Health Care–Associated Transmission of Hepatitis B and C Viruses

Guest Editor

BANDAR AL KNAWY, MD, FRCPC

CLINICS IN LIVER DISEASE

www.liver.theclinics.com

Consulting Editor
NORMAN GITLIN, MD

February 2010 • Volume 14 • Number 1

SAUNDERS an imprint of ELSEVIER, Inc.

W.B. SAUNDERS COMPANY

A Division of Elsevier Inc.

1600 John F. Kennedy Boulevard, Suite 1800 • Philadelphia, PA 19103-2899

http://www.theclinics.com

CLINICS IN LIVER DISEASE Volume 14, Number 1
February 2010 ISSN 1089-3261, ISBN-13: 978-1-4377-1915-4

Editor: Kerry Holland
Developmental Editor: Donald Mumford

Clinics in Liver Disease (ISSN 1089-3261) is published quarterly by Elsevier Inc., 360 Park Avenue South, New York, NY 10010-1710. Months of issue are February, May, August, and November. Business and Editorial Offices: 1600 John F. Kennedy Blvd., Ste. 1800, Philadelphia, PA 19103-2899. Customer Service Office: 3251 Riverport Lane, Maryland Heights, MO 63043. Periodicals postage paid at New York, NY and additional mailing offices. Subscription prices are $235.00 per year (U.S. individuals), $118.00 per year (U.S. student/resident), $340.00 per year (U.S. institutions), $311.00 per year (foreign individuals), $163.00 per year (foreign student/ resident), $409.00 per year (foreign instituitions), $271.00 per year (Canadian individuals), $163.00 per year (Canadian student/resident), and $409.00 per year (Canadian institutions). Foreign air speed delivery is included in all *Clinics* subscription prices. All prices are subject to change without notice. **POSTMASTER:** Send address changes to *Clinics in Liver Disease*, Elsevier Health Sciences Division, Subscription Customer Service, 3251 Riverport Lane, Maryland Heights, MO 63043. **Customer Service: Telephone: 1-800-654-2452 (U.S. and Canada); 314-447-8871 (outside U.S. and Canada). Fax: 314-447-8029. E-mail: journalscustomer service-usa@elsevier.com (for print support); journalsonlinesupport-usa@elsevier.com (for online support).**

Reprints. For copies of 100 or more of articles in this publication, please contact the Commercial Reprints Department, Elsevier Inc., 360 Park Avenue South, New York, NY 10010-1710. Tel.: 212-633-3812; Fax: 212-462-1935; E-mail: reprints@elsevier.com.

Clinics in Liver Disease is covered in *MEDLINE/PubMed (Index Medicus)*.

Printed and bound in the United Kingdom
Transferred to Digital Print 2011

Contributors

CONSULTING EDITOR

NORMAN M. GITLIN, MD, FRCP (LONDON), FRCPE (EDINBURGH), FACG, FACP
Formerly, Professor of Medicine, Chief of Hepatology, Emory University; Currently, Consultant, Gastroenterology Associates, Atlanta, Georgia

GUEST EDITOR

BANDAR AL KNAWY, MD, FRCPC
Consultant, Division of Gastroenterology & Hepatology, Department of Medicine, King Abdulaziz Medical City, National Guard Health Affairs, Riyadh, Saudi Arabia

AUTHORS

MARY ANNE BOBINSKI, BA, JD, LLM
Dean and Professor, Faculty of Law, University of British Columbia, Vancouver, British Columbia, Canada

ABIGAIL L. CARLSON, BA
Research Associate, Department of Hospital Epidemiology and Infection Control, The Johns Hopkins Hospital, Baltimore, Maryland

MICHAEL B. EDMOND, MD, MPH, MPA
Chair, Division of Infectious Diseases, Virginia Commonwealth University Medical Center; Professor of Internal Medicine, Epidemiology and Community Health; Hospital Epidemiologist, Virginia Commonwealth University School of Medicine, Richmond, Virginia

FABRIZIO FABRIZI, MD
Staff Nephrologist, Division of Nephrology, Maggiore Hospital, IRCCS Foundation, Milano, Italy; Research Associate, Center for Liver Diseases, School of Medicine, University of Miami, Miami, Florida

AHMED GOMAA, MD, ScD, MSPH
Division of Surveillance Hazard Evaluation and Health Studies, National Institute for Occupational Safety and Health, Centers for Disease Control and Prevention, Cincinnati, Ohio

DAVID K. HENDERSON, MD
Deputy Director for Clinical Care; Hospital Epidemiology Service, NIH Clinical Center, Bethesda, Maryland

SCOTT D. HOLMBERG, MD, MPH
Chief, Epidemiology and Surveillance Branch, Division of Viral Hepatitis, National Center for HIV, Hepatitis, TB and STD Prevention (NCHHSTP), Centers for Disease Control and Prevention (CDC), Atlanta, Georgia

DONALD M. JENSEN, MD
Professor of Medicine, Director, Center for Liver Diseases, Department of Medicine, University of Chicago Medical Center, Chicago, Illinois

ANGELA K. LARAMIE, MPH
Sharps Injury Surveillance Project, Occupational Health Surveillance Program, Massachusetts Department of Public Health, Boston, Massachusetts

TARANISIA MacCANNELL, MSc, PhD
Division of Healthcare Quality Promotion, Centers for Disease Control and Prevention, Atlanta, Georgia

ANURAG MAHESHWARI, MD
Institute of Digestive Health and Liver Diseases, Mercy Medical Center, Baltimore, Maryland

PAUL MARTIN, MD
Professor of Medicine and Chief, Division of Hepatology, Department of Medicine, Center for Liver Diseases, Miller School of Medicine, University of Miami, Miami, Florida

ANGELA MICHELIN, MPH
Hospital Epidemiology Service, NIH Clinical Center, Bethesda, Maryland

PRITI R. PATEL, MD, MPH
Division of Healthcare Quality Promotion, Prevention and Response Branch, Centers for Disease Control and Prevention, Atlanta, Georgia

TRISH M. PERL, MD, MSc
Director, Department of Hospital Epidemiology and Infection Control, The Johns Hopkins Hospital; Professor of Medicine and Pathology, Division of Infectious Diseases, Department of Medicine, Johns Hopkins University School of Medicine; Professor of Epidemiology, Department of Epidemiology, Johns Hopkins University Bloomberg School of Public Health, Baltimore, Maryland

JOSEPH F. PERZ, DrPH, MA
Division of Healthcare Quality Promotion, Prevention and Response Branch, Centers for Disease Control and Prevention, Atlanta, Georgia

MELISSA K. SCHAEFER, MD
Division of Healthcare Quality Promotion, Prevention and Response Branch, Centers for Disease Control and Prevention; Epidemic Intelligence Service, Office of Workforce and Career Development, Centers for Disease Control and Prevention, Atlanta, Georgia

BO SHEN, MD
Digestive Disease Institute, Cleveland Clinic, Cleveland, Ohio

MITCHELL L. SHIFFMAN, MD
Bon Secours Health System, Liver Institute of Virginia, Richmond, Virginia

MICHAEL P. STEVENS, MD
Fellow in Infectious Diseases and Hospital Epidemiology, Division of Infectious Diseases, Virginia Commonwealth University Medical Center, Richmond, Virginia

HELEN S. TE, MD
Associate Professor of Medicine, Medical Director of Liver Transplantation, Center for Liver Diseases, Department of Medicine, University of Chicago Medical Center, Chicago, Illinois

NICOLA D. THOMPSON, PhD, MS
Division of Viral Hepatitis, Centers for Disease Control and Prevention, Epidemiology and Surveillance Branch, Atlanta, Georgia

PAUL J. THULUVATH, MD, FRCP
Professor of Surgery (Transplantation) and Medicine, Department of Surgery and Medicine, Georgetown University School of Medicine, Washington, DC; Medical Director, Institute for Digestive and Liver Diseases, Mercy Medical Center, Baltimore, Maryland

HAO WU, MB
Department of Gastroenterology, Zhongshan Hospital, Fudan University, Shanghai, China

FARIBA S. YOUNAI, DDS
Clinical Professor, Department of Oral Medicine & Orofacial Pain; Vice-Chair, Division of Oral Biology and Medicine, UCLA School of Dentistry, Los Angeles, California

Contents

mutations; molecular clock analyses of the short-term evolution of HCV; and analyses of clades and surface antigen polymorphisms of HBV. However, for most epidemiologists molecular epidemiology of viral hepatitis usually refers to studies of gene-sequence homology in HBV or HCV recovered from people in the community or an institution that allows better characterization and assignment of related clusters of infection.

and develop long-lasting immunity. In contrast, the vast majority of patients who develop chronic HBV have minimal symptoms and do not develop jaundice after becoming infected with HBV. These patients will frequently remain undiagnosed for years or decades. Approximately 1% of persons with acute HBV develop acute liver failure. Preventing acute HBV with vaccination is the best treatment. Although universal vaccination is now administered to newborns in many countries, the majority of adults have not been vaccinated and remain at risk. Because the majority of patients with acute HBV resolve this infection spontaneously, treatment with an oral anti-HBV agent is not necessary. However, the use of an oral anti-HBV agent is not unreasonable to use in a patient who is developing acute liver failure from severe acute HBV.

THE CLINICS ARE NOW AVAILABLE ONLINE!

Access your subscription at:
www.theclinics.com

Preface

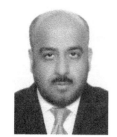

Bandar Al Knawy, MD, FRCPC
Guest Editor

Worldwide, a number of health care transmission outbreaks of infectious diseases, particularly hepatitis, in the past decade indicate startling evidence of an ongoing transmission of hepatitis in a health care setting.

News reports describing the disease as the "giant that sleeps no longer" and outbreaks that represent the "tip of an iceberg," as reported by the Centers for Disease Control and Prevention, have put unsafe injection practices in health care in the spotlight. The specific outbreaks have been attributed to the reuse of syringes on multiple patients and by drawing medication from multidose vials. The disregard for basic safety injection practices that led to these incidents presented a grave threat to patient safety, outrage, and mistrust in the health care system. This also prompted health officials in various states to enact public health legislation for the prevention of similar situations.

This issue of *Clinics in Liver Disease* offers the latest information regarding the transmission of hepatitis viruses in various health care settings. The articles address the subject of patient safety, which targets health care professionals, gastroenterologists, hepatologists, oncologists, and dentists and discusses ways for all health care workers to adopt and share a variety of best practices to prevent the adverse event of hepatitis transmission.

Well-known experts in liver disease, infection control, and medical practice in a legal setting have been assembled to produce a comprehensive and concise edition that highlights the latest information regarding hepatitis B and C transmission in health care. The articles provide an overview of the most important topics: molecular epidemiology; outbreak reports; the transmission in hemodialysis, endoscopy, dental, and oncology patients; management; legal aspects; and the infection prevention measures to reduce the risk of needless exposure of patients to these blood-borne pathogens.

Creating a safe, reliable, and high-performance environment in health care facilities requires a unique combination of strategies and unrelenting determination for strict enforcement of infection control practices. Prevention of health care–associated

Clin Liver Dis 14 (2010) xiii–xiv
doi:10.1016/j.cld.2009.11.014
1089-3261/10/$ – see front matter
liver.theclinics.com

transmission of hepatitis involves comprehensive measures, such as better surveillance, education, and management. I hope that you enjoy reading this issue and add it to your collection of the *Clinics in Liver Disease*.

Bandar Al Knawy, MD, FRCPC
Division of Gastroenterology & Hepatology
Department of Medicine
King Abdulaziz Medical City
National Guard Health Affairs
Riyadh, Saudi Arabia

E-mail address:
knawyb@ngha.med.sa

Epidemiology of Hepatitis B and C Viruses: A Global Overview

Helen S. Te, MD[a],*, Donald M. Jensen, MD[b]

KEYWORDS

- Epidemiology • Hepatitis B • Hepatitis C
- Global • Endemicity

The pace of therapeutic advances in the treatment of chronic viral hepatitis, such as hepatitis B and hepatitis C, has accelerated significantly in the past decade. The hepatitis B virus (HBV) vaccination program also expanded its coverage globally, and limited treatment options in the past have given way to a multitude of effective drugs for HBV. On the other hand, blood product safety has become increasingly optimized, and improvements in the preparation of existing antiviral medications and better understanding of viral kinetics during therapy have paved the way for improved treatment success rates in hepatitis C virus (HCV) infection. In addition, several novel agents for both diseases are under active investigation and are expected to expand the treatment opportunities in the future. To be able to consider the appropriate population for diagnosis and treatment of HBV or HCV infection, the changing epidemiology and transmission patterns of these diseases merit a revisit. Here, the authors review the prevalence, disease burden, genotype distribution, and transmission patterns of HBV and HCV in the 6 World Health Organization (WHO) regions (**Fig. 1**) around the world.

HEPATITIS B
Worldwide Prevalence and Disease Burden

HBV is a DNA virus that infects only humans and is highly contagious, more so than HCV or human immunodeficiency virus (HIV). HBV is transmitted by parenteral or

[a] Liver Transplantation, Center for Liver Diseases, Department of Medicine, University of Chicago Medical Center, 5841 South Maryland Avenue, MC 7120, Chicago, IL 60637, USA
[b] Center for Liver Diseases, Department of Medicine, University of Chicago Medical Center, 5841 South Maryland Avenue, MC 7120, Chicago, IL 60637, USA
* Corresponding author.
E-mail address: hte@medicine.bsd.uchicago.edu (H.S. Te).

Clin Liver Dis 14 (2010) 1–21
doi:10.1016/j.cld.2009.11.009
1089-3261/10/$ – see front matter © 2010 Elsevier Inc. All rights reserved.

liver.theclinics.com

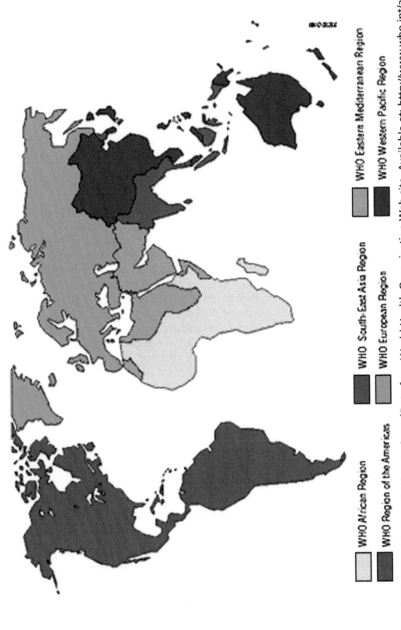

Fig. 1. Map of World Health Organization regions. (*Data from* World Health Organization Web site. Available at: http://www.who.int/about/regions/en/index.html. Accessed March 4, 2009.)

WHO African Region
WHO Region of the Americas
WHO South-East Asia Region
WHO European Region
WHO Eastern Mediterranean Region
WHO Western Pacific Region

mucosal exposure to infected blood and serous fluid, where its concentration is the highest, and body fluids such as semen and vaginal fluid. Common routes of infection include mother to infant, child to child, unsafe injection practices, sexual contact, and blood transfusions.

Approximately 5% of all acute HBV infections progress to chronic infection, and the risk of progression from an acute to chronic phase is inversely proportional to age. Up to 90% of infants who acquire HBV infection from their mothers at birth become chronically infected. Among children who become infected with HBV between 1 year and 5 years of age, 30% to 50% become chronically infected. In adults, chronic HBV infection results in 5% of acute cases.

The implementation of universal hepatitis vaccination for infants in most countries has lowered the prevalence of HBV over the past decades. As of the end of 2007, HBV vaccine has been introduced to a total of 171 countries and an estimated 65% of the world's population, as compared with 3% in 1992. The coverage is highest in the Americas at 88%, while it is at 69% in Africa and 30% in the South-East Asia.[1] Universal vaccination has been expected to reduce HBV prevalence, but in some parts of the world, newer estimates have been higher than previous due to the use of more sensitive assays. Nevertheless, the global burden of HBV remains high, with about 2 billion people exposed worldwide and about 350 million individuals with chronic infection who may be at risk for complications of liver cancer or progressive liver disease. Hepatitis B is estimated to be the cause of 30% of cirrhosis and 53% of hepatocellular carcinoma (HCC) worldwide.[2] An estimated 600,000 deaths each year can be attributed to acute or chronic HBV infection.[3]

About 45% of HBV infected individuals live in areas with a high prevalence of 8% or more, where the lifetime risk of infection is more than 60%, typically occurring in infancy and early childhood. These individuals have a high risk of chronicity, which in turn increases the risk for the development of hepatocellular carcinoma and complications of cirrhosis. In China, South-East Asia, most of Africa, most Pacific Islands, parts of the Middle East, and the Amazon Basin, the prevalence is as high as 8% to 15%. Forty-three percent of infected individuals live in areas with an intermediate prevalence of 2% to 7%, where the lifetime risk of infection is 20% to 60%, typically occurring across all age groups. These areas include south-central and south-west Asia, eastern and southern Europe, Russia, as well as Central and South America. The remaining 12% live in low prevalence areas of less than 2%, where the lifetime risk of infection is less than 20%, typically occurring in adulthood. These low prevalence areas include the United States, Western Europe, and Australia (**Fig. 2**).[3,4]

Genotypes

There are 8 genotypes, A to H, described for HBV, which have a distinctive geographic distribution. Genotype A is more prevalent in northwestern Europe, North America, India, and sub-Saharan Africa, and less commonly in some regions of South America. Genotypes B and C are endemic to Asia, while genotype D predominates in the Mediterranean region and Eastern Europe, although it can also be found all over the world.[5] Genotype E is characteristic of Western Africa, genotype F in South America, and genotype H in Central America. Lastly, genotype G has been reported in France, Germany, Central America, Mexico, and the United States.[5–11] Individual countries and its local regions, as well individual population groups at risk, may harbor specific genotypes at varying prevalence rates.[5]

At the present time, HBV genotypes may have clinical significance in terms of treatment outcomes, with patients infected with genotype A and B having better response to interferon than those with genotype C and D.[12] The association of specific HBV

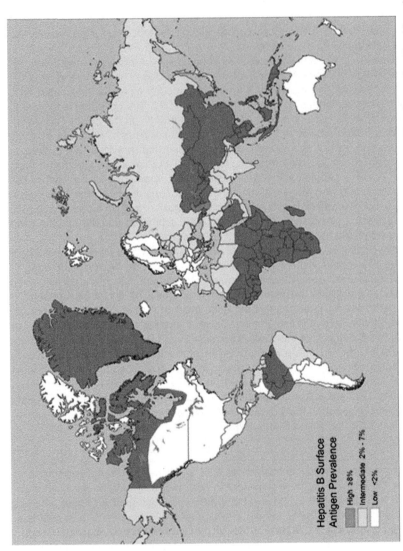

Fig. 2. Geographic distribution of hepatitis B infection worldwide, 2006. (*Data from* Center for Disease Control. Travelers' health: yellow book. Atlanta, GA: U.S. Department of Health and Human Services, CDC; 2008. Available at: http://wwwn.cdc.gov/travel/yellowBookCh4-HepB.aspx#363. Accessed March 4, 2009.)

genotype with disease progression and risk for HCC is variable, depending on the country where it is studied. Genotype C, for example, portends a more severe disease in Taiwan whereas genotype B is associated with the development of HCC in young, noncirrhotic patients; however, genotype B has a relatively good prognosis in Japan and China, with no strong association to HCC. In India, genotype D is associated with more severe liver disease and HCC in young patients than genotype A.[13]

Americas

The WHO Americas region comprises 35 member states in North America, South and Central Americas, as well as Mexico. Hepatitis B prevalence in the Americas needs to be considered in the context of 2 distinct subgroups: North America (United States and Canada) with its low prevalence, and South and Central Americas with their heterogeneous but significantly higher prevalence.

North America
Based on blood donor studies, the overall prevalence of hepatitis B surface antigen (HBsAg) carriers is 0.2% in the United States.[14] However, the Centers for Disease Control and Prevention (CDC) estimated that 1.25 million Americans or nearly 0.5% of the population are chronic carriers of HBV, and an additional 5000 to 8000 become chronically infected each year.[15] The incidence of HBV also varies greatly amongst the American population, being highest in immigrants or refugees from areas of high endemicity, followed by the Native Alaskans[16] and blacks. Among the whites, Hispanics had a higher rate of infection than non-Hispanics. The highest rates of infection occur in individuals aged 20 to 39 years.[4] Because infection in childhood tend to be asymptomatic, less than 5% of acute HBV in this age group are reported to the CDC. In addition to childhood infections, 20,000 infants are estimated to be born to HBsAg-positive mothers per year,[17] with the prevalence being higher in urban settings.[18]

The incidence of reported acute HBV peaked in the mid-1980s at 26,000 cases per year, and declined significantly during 1990 to 2004, with 4758 cases reported in 2006.[15] This incidence coincided with the increased vaccine coverage initiatives in 1991, targeting prenatal screening of infected pregnant women and universal vaccination of infants, adolescents, and adults at risk for HBV, leading to lower rates of infection among children and adolescents.[4] About 200 to 300 Americans die of fulminant infection each year, and approximately 25% of HBsAg carriers develop progressive disease that often leads to complications such as cirrhosis or HCC. An estimated 3000 to 4000 individuals die of HBV-related cirrhosis and an estimated 1000 to 1500 individuals die of HBV-related HCC in the United States per year.[4]

In Canada, the incidence rate of acute HBV was estimated to be 2.0 cases per 100,000 population (approximately 700 cases a year) in 2006.[19] The rate is higher among males than females, and peaks at the age of 30 to 39 years (4.8 cases per 100,000).[20] The prevalence of HBV has been estimated at 0.7% to 0.9% of the population,[19] except for the immigrant populations and the Inuit, in whom the prevalence is higher at 7.4% and 6.9%, respectively.[21]

The routes of HBV transmission are similar in the United States and Canada, with adult horizontal transmission being the most common, except for the recent immigrants, Native Alaskans, and northern Native Canadians, where vertical and childhood horizontal transmissions still predominate.[4,21]

South and Central America
The WHO South and Central Americas region includes 32 countries in this region along with Mexico. Although HBV is considered to be highly prevalent in this region, there is

a complex pattern of prevalence not only amongst the countries but also within them. The estimated HBsAg seroprevalence ranges from 0.5% to 3%, with the total number of HBsAg carriers approaching 11 million.[22–24] The highest prevalence of up to 8% is among the native populations of the western Amazon basin, which includes Brazil, Colombia, Peru, and Venezuela. The prevalence decreases with increasing distance from this area, with Chile, Uruguay, Paraguay and Argentina having the lowest HBsAg prevalence. In the middle are Haiti, the Dominican Republic, and Honduras, with an HBsAg prevalence of about 3%.[25] In a more systematic epidemiologic study covering 6 countries (Argentina, Brazil, Chile, Dominican Republic, Mexico, Venezuela), the Dominican Republic was noted to have the highest prevalence of HBV core antibody (21.4%), followed by Brazil (7.9%), Venezuela (3.2%), and Argentina (2.1%). The lowest prevalence was in Mexico (1.4%) and Chile (0.6%).[23,24] Based on the lowest annual estimate of 140,000 acute HBV infections in Latin America each year, about 8,000 to 15,000 chronic HBsAg carriers are expected, amongst whom more than 4000 are expected to follow a chronic active infection course. Up to 60,000 cases of cirrhosis and 3000 cases of HCC have been linked to HBV infection in this region.[26]

The routes of HBV transmission in South and Central America are highly variable. The highest prevalence has been reported to be at the 20- to 40-year-old age group, supporting adult horizontal transmission as the most common route of infection, through either sexual or parenteral means. In addition, cultural practices such as tattooing also contribute to the risk. However, vertical transmission and childhood horizontal transmission play larger roles in areas of high endemicity such as the Amazon Basin.[26,27] In the isolated Yanomano communities of the Upper Orinoco Basin, majority (75%) of the HBsAg carriers who were also hepatitis B e antigen (HBeAg) positive were mostly women of childbearing age, and the prevalence of HBsAg in children aged 1 to 4 years was 33% amidst a hepatitis B core antibody (HBcore Ab) prevalence of 66%.[28,29]

Africa

The WHO Africa region covers all of sub-Saharan Africa and Algeria, comprising 46 member states. The burden of HBV in Africa is difficult to assess due to underreporting and inaccurate records. The estimated HBsAg seroprevalence ranges from 5% to 20%, with the total number of HBsAg carriers approaching an astounding 40 to 58 million.[22–24] As many as 70% to 95% of the adult population have markers of past HBV exposure.[30] Western Africa is an area of very high HBV endemicity, with HBsAg prevalence being more than 10% in Gambia and Senegal. In addition, HCC is a major public health problem in this region, and is the most frequent cause of death in males and the second most frequent in females.[31] In Gambia, 57% of HCC cases were attributed to HBV infection; these occurred more commonly in males in a 5:1 ratio to females and at a median of 40 years of age.[32] In South Africa, ethnic groups have variable prevalence rates of HBV markers. The rate is highest in blacks in rural areas who have HBsAg rates from 7.5% to 14% and markers of prior exposure from 76% to 98%. Chronic HBsAg carriage and markers of HBV infection are detected in 0.2% and 5% of whites and East Indians, and in 5.3% and 50% of the Chinese population.[33]

The route of transmission in this region seems to be childhood horizontal transmission. In Senegal, where the endemicity is very high, 59% of children younger than 5 years had markers of prior HBV exposure.[34] The risk of infection increased steadily in the child's first years of life, and the HBsAg prevalence is 6% at 6 months of age and 13% at 2 years of age. Markers of previous HBV infection were detected in 30% after 2 years of age and in more than 90% after age 10 years.[35] Although vertical transmission occurs,[36] the lower rate of infection in infancy than in older children supported horizontal transmission as the cause of endemicity.[37,38] Transmission is believed to be via saliva or blood exposure percutaneously through wounds or bites.[39] Sexual transmission in adults also occur but a lower rate, with HBsAg being detected in14% and markers of previous HBV exposure being present in 89% of young sexually active adults attending a sexually transmitted disease clinic.[40] Unlike South-East Asia, perinatal transmission seems to be less common in this region,[41] with HBsAg prevalence of 4.3% to 5.4% in pregnant women.[42,43] The introduction of HBV vaccine in Gambia in 1986 and in South Africa in 1995 have decreased the risk of vertical transmission and provided protection against HBsAg carriage.[44,45]

Eastern Mediterranean

The WHO Eastern Mediterranean region consists of 21 member states located in North Africa and the Middle East, as well as Pakistan. The WHO estimate of HBsAg prevalence in this region ranged from 1% to 10% in 1997. Throughout the region, transmission occurs through childhood horizontal and adult horizontal routes and, less commonly, vertical routes.[22]

In Egypt, the estimated HBsAg prevalence is 6.7% among healthy population-based studies, accounting for about 350 million carriers. Adults have a higher prevalence of 8% compared with children at 1.6%, most likely a result of the introduction of HBV vaccines for children in 1992.[46] HBsAg prevalence is higher in males than in females, despite a comparable prevalence of HBV markers in both, suggesting that women may be more likely to clear the infection than men. Before HBV vaccines were implemented in the 1980s, the peak of HBsAg prevalence occurred in the age groups 14 to 18 years in Upper Egypt and 39 to 48 years in Lower Egypt, both supporting a late childhood and adult horizontal means of transmission.[47] Before the vaccine, HBV was the dominant disease associated with HCC in Egypt,[48] but the introduction of the vaccine has led to a lower overall prevalence of HBV among HCC cases at about 25%. Childhood immunization coverage for HBV in Egypt is estimated at 95% to 100%, making it highly likely that HBV prevalence and its associated complications will decline over the next decades.[46]

In Pakistan, the estimated prevalence of HBV in the general population is estimated at 2.5% or 5.6 million individuals, based on a seroprevalence study conducted by the Pakistan Medical Research Council.[49] However, an HBsAg prevalence of 3.3% has been reported in blood donors[50] and of 2.9% in young military men.[51] In Iran, the prevalence of HBsAg is 2.3%, and a history of surgery and imprisonment are identified as risk factors for the infection.[52]

Europe

The WHO Europe region extends from Iceland to Turkey and includes Israel and the former Soviet Union, covering 53 member states. The prevalence of HBsAg in the general population is heterogeneous in this region, with Northern Europe having the lowest prevalence rate of less than 0.1%, Western Europe having the intermediate prevalence rates of 0.1% to 0.5%, and an overall higher prevalence rate of 2.4% (<0.5% to >5%) in Southern and Eastern Europe.[53] Specific countries demonstrate variable prevalence rates as well, with intermediate to high rates in Turkey (8%) and Romania (6%), intermediate rates in Bulgaria (4%), Latvia (2%), and Greece (2%), and lower rates in the Slovak Republic, Poland, Czech Republic, Belgium, Lithuania, Italy, and Germany (0.5%–1.5%). The Netherlands, Estonia, Hungary, Slovenia, and Norway have less than 0.5% prevalence, although Estonia has a high incidence rate.[11] Over the past decade, there has been a steady decline in reported cases of hepatitis B in the European Union and the European Economic Arc/European Free Trade Association member states and countries, from 6.7 cases per 100,000 population in 1995 to 1.5 cases per 100,000 population in 2005.[11] The highest incidence of HBV is in the age group 25 to 44 years (2.98 cases per 100,000) followed by the 15 to 24 year age group (2.49 cases per 100,000). HBV is more common in males (1.33 cases per 100,000) than females (0.58 cases per 100,000).[54] In 2005, Iceland reported the highest incidence at 13.5 cases per 100,000, followed by Bulgaria at 12.42 cases per 100,000. There was a steady decline in reported HBV cases in almost all countries by 2007, with Bulgaria reporting 9.89 cases per 100,000 (Iceland had no data for this year), except for Austria where the incidence appears to be on the rise.[55] Despite an influx of immigrants from highly endemic Africa to Italy in the past decade, the overall prevalence of HBV in Northern Italy is practically unchanged.[56]

The mode of transmission is dependent on the prevalence of HBV in the specific places, and include heterosexual and male homosexual activity, intravenous drug use (IVDU), perinatal exposure, and close household contacts.[22] In countries with intermediate to high endemicity, vertical transmission and horizontal transmission within infected households are the most common routes of infection, whereas in low endemic areas, IVDU and sexual activity are the predominant means. In the Netherlands, sexual transmission is the most frequent means of transmission,[57] whereas in Central and Eastern Europe nosocomial infection such as blood transfusion and medical procedures account for up to 60% of HBV infections in adults and 80% in children.[58,59] However, vertical transmission and childhood horizontal transmission are important in maintaining the high endemicity in the former Soviet Union.[22] Today, strict screening of blood, vaccination, and improved sanitation standards have all led to a declining trend of HBV prevalence in most countries.[22,56,59] In Italy, the incidence of acute HBV decreased by 50% from 1988 to 1994, corresponding to an estimated 90% vaccination coverage rate in infants and adolescents in 1994.[60–62]

South-East Asia

The South-East Asia region extends from India to Indonesia, and covers a total of 11 member states that include India, Indonesia, and Thailand. The WHO estimated HBsAg prevalence in this region was 1% to 10% in 1997, with about 130 million carriers.[22] However, introduction of a more global childhood immunization program has undoubtedly led to declining prevalence rates in most of these countries.

In Thailand, the prevalence of HBV carriers has declined in 1987 to 1991, from 8.2% to 6.5% among blood donors and 6.6% to 5.2% among students.[63] Among children younger than 15 years, the overall prevalence of HBV carriers is much lower at 0.55% with a corresponding HBsAb prevalence of 58.5%.[64] As with other high endemicity areas, the infection is more common among males than females, with a 3:1 male to female ratio among blood donors who were studied.[65] The highest prevalence is reported in the young age group of 15 to 40 years.[63,65–67] Vertical and horizontal spread, both in childhood and adulthood, are the predominant means of transmission in Thailand.

In India, the average prevalence of HBsAg is 4%,[22,68] accounting for more than 40 to 50 million carriers.[69] HBsAg is detected in 33% to 75% of individuals diagnosed with chronic liver disease and in 56% to 70% of individuals with cirrhosis. The reported prevalence ranges from 2.5% to 7.7% in various states in the country,[70] and an increasing prevalence is observed from north to south.[68] However, an extensive review by the Indian National Association for the study of Liver Diseases reported a consensus figure of 4.7% as the prevalence of HBsAg nationwide.[71] Males are more frequently infected with HBV than females.[72] Transmission includes vertical means and adult horizontal means, but is mostly through childhood horizontal means due to the suboptimal hygiene and crowded living conditions.[68] Since 2002, HBV vaccine has been implemented in broader areas of India, but further expansion of coverage still is necessary.

Western Pacific

The highest endemicity for HBV in the world is in the Western Pacific region, where HBsAg prevalence is from 5% to 35% among the 37 countries, except for Australia (non-Aborigine population), New Zealand, and Japan, where the carriage rate is lower at less than 2%.[73] This region is home to 28% of the global population, but harbors 45% (150 million) of chronic HBsAg carriers and accounts for more than half of the HBV-related deaths throughout the world. The north and central Asian countries such as China, South Korea, and Taiwan as well as the Philippines have HBsAg prevalence rates between 10% and 12%.[22]

The means of transmission is largely vertical and also childhood horizontal, which results in a high rate of chronicity.[22] In the Philippines, HBsAg prevalence peaks in the 2- to 9-year-old group in some areas, but others have the peak in the 30- to 49-year-old group,[74] indicating both early life and adulthood transmission. Sexual transmission, IVDU, and poor sterilization of medical equipment are potential ways for adult horizontal transmission.[75]

In Taiwan, 40% to 50% of HBsAg positive women of childbearing age had active HBV replication states as indicated by a positive HBeAg, suggesting perinatal transmission as a means of endemicity.[76] However, the most important mode of transmission is believed to be childhood horizontal, accounting for 50% to 80% of HBV infection.[73,77] Here, HCC is strongly linked to HBV infection, but the association is even more pronounced in children in whom HBsAg was present in almost 100% of HCC cases, as compared with adults who had HBsAg positivity in 70% to 80%. The nationwide HBV vaccination program launched in 1984 has reduced the HBsAg carrier rate from 10% to 1% in Taiwanese children,[78,79] and has consequently reduced the average annual incidence of HCC in children aged 6 to 14 from 0.70 cases per 100,000 in the early 1980s to 0.36 cases per 100,000 a decade later.[78]

HEPATITIS C
Worldwide Prevalence and Disease Burden

Hepatitis C is an RNA virus known to infect humans and chimpanzees, causing a similar disease in these 2 species. HCV is the most common cause of transfusion-related hepatitis, and is one of the leading causes of end-stage-liver disease requiring liver transplantation in the United States. HCV is transmitted most efficiently by parenteral means, particularly with large or repeated exposure to infected blood products or transplantation of infected tissue or organ grafts, and IVDU. Less frequently, it can be transmitted by mucosal exposures to blood or serum-derived fluids through perinatal or sexual means.[80]

The relative mutability of the HCV genome has been blamed for its high propensity to cause chronic infection. About 80% of new infections progress on to chronic infection, with cirrhosis developing in about 20% after 20 to 30 years, resulting in increased risk for liver-related complications and HCC. The high mutability of the HCV genome and limited knowledge in the protective immune response following infection has hindered progress in vaccine development. For this reason, no vaccine is available against HCV.[81]

The WHO estimated global prevalence of HCV infection was 3% or 170 million individuals in 1999. The prevalence was higher in some countries in Africa (5.3% or 31.9 million), the eastern Mediterranean (4.6% or 21.3 million), South-East Asia (2.15% or 32.3 million) and the Western Pacific (3.9% or 62.2 million), as compared with some countries in the Americas (1.7% or 13.1 million) and Europe (1.03% or 8.9 million).[81] In 2004, the Global Burden of Hepatitis C Working Group, serving as a consultant to the WHO, estimated the global prevalence to be slightly lower at 2.2% or 130 million individuals. The lowest HCV prevalence of 0.01% to 0.1% is from countries in the United Kingdom and Scandinavia, while the highest prevalence of 15% to 20% is from Egypt (**Fig. 3**).[82] Hepatitis C is estimated to be the cause of 27% of cirrhosis and 25% of HCC worldwide.[2]

Genotypes

There are 11 HCV genotypes (genotypes 1 to 11), many subtypes (a, b, c, and so forth), and about 100 different strains (1, 2, 3, and so forth) based on the sequence heterogeneity of the HCV genome. Genotypes 1 to 3 are widely distributed globally, with genotypes 1a and 1b accounting for 60% of infections worldwide. Genotype 1a is predominantly located in Northern Europe and North America, while genotype 1b is predominantly found in Southern and Eastern Europe and Japan. Genotype 2 is less common than genotype 1, and is found more in Europe than in North America. Genotype 3 is endemic in South-East Asia, and genotype 4 is characteristic for the Middle East, Egypt, and central Africa. Genotype 5 is almost exclusively found in South Africa, and genotypes 6 to 11 are mostly distributed in Asia.[80,83–86]

The impact of viral genotype in the pathogenesis of liver disease remains a subject of controversy, but the influence of the genotype in the response to interferon-based therapy is established. Genotype 1 is generally associated with a poorer response to therapy while genotypes 2 and 3 have a more favorable response. Genotype 4 seems to have an intermediate response.[86,87]

Americas

In the United States, the prevalence of HCV has been estimated from the National Health and Nutrition Examination Survey (NHANES), with the most recent one conducted by the CDC from 1999 to 2002. The overall incidence of HCV exposure as detected by serum HCV antibody is 1.6% or 4.1 million individuals, but the estimated prevalence of chronic infection as measured by serum HCV RNA is at 1.3% or 3.2 million individuals. The survey, however, failed to assess the homeless or incarcerated, so the true prevalence is probably higher. The infection is more common in men (2.1%) than women (1.1%), and has a higher prevalence in non-Hispanic blacks (3%) than in non-Hispanic whites (91.5%) and Mexican Americans (1.3%). The peak age group affected is 45 to 49 years, representing an upward shift of the peak age group of 35 to 39 years in the previous NHANES III study in 1988 to 1994. Most individuals with HCV were born between 1945 and 1964.[88]

Before the implementation of universal screening of blood donors in 1992, the predominant mode of transmission was exposure to infected blood and blood products. At present, IVDU and high-risk sexual exposures account for most HCV transmission.[82] The enhanced screening of blood products has led to a decline of the estimated incidence of acute hepatitis C from 180,000 in the mid-1980s to an estimated 19,000 in 2006.[15] HCV is estimated to cause 8000 to 10,000 deaths per year related to liver complications and HCC.[82]

In Canada, the estimated prevalence of HCV infection is about 0.8%, or 210,000 to 275,000 individuals. The national surveillance system, Enhanced Hepatitis Strain

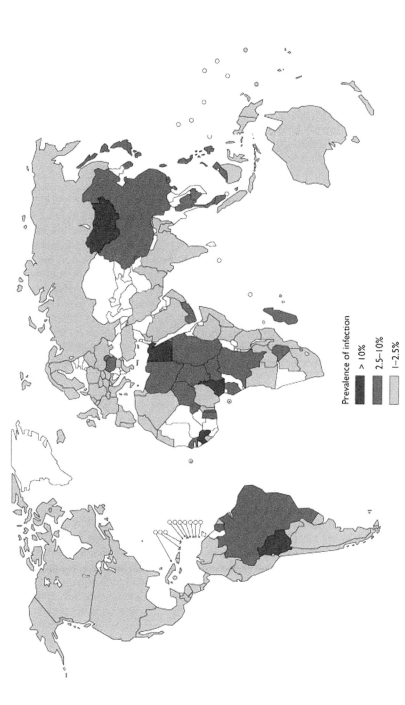

Fig. 3. Geographic distribution of hepatitis C infection worldwide, 2007. (*Data from* World Health Organization. Internal travel and health. Available at: http://www.who.int/ith/maps/hepatitisc2007.jpg. Accessed March 11, 2009.)

Surveillance System, reported a decline in new HCV infections from 3.3 cases per 100,000 in 1998 to 2.1 cases per 100,000 in 2004. The peak age group affected was 15 to 39 years of age.[89] The declining incidence reflects the reduction in transmission via blood and blood products with modern blood screening procedures, and injection drug use has become the major means of transmission, being associated with at least half of new HCV infections.[90] Sexual transmission of HCV is uncommon.

In Latin America, the overall prevalence of HCV antibody is estimated to be 1.23%. However, the prevalence of HCV antibody in blood donors varies from region to region, with an estimate of 0.2% to 0.5% in Chile, 0.8% to 2.8% in south-east Brazil, and 1.7% to 3.4% in north-east Brazil.[91] In Mexico, the prevalence of HCV exposure is estimated at 0.0% to 2.7% in non–blood donor asymptomatic individuals. Here, the main risk factors are blood transfusion, unprotected sex, or multiple sexual partners.[92,93]

Africa

The WHO region of Africa has the highest estimated prevalence of HCV at 5.3% or 31.9 million.[81] Central Africa is the most endemic at 6%, followed by west Africa at 2.4%, while southern and east Africa have the lowest estimate at 1.6%.[94] In Central Africa, Burundi and Cameroon have the highest prevalence of 11.3% and 13.8%, respectively. The prevalence increases with age, with the highest rate being reported in the age group older than 40 years. Inconsistent screening procedures for blood donors make blood transfusion a major means of acquisition of HCV infection, as evidenced by a high HCV prevalence in sickle cell patients who have received multiple blood transfusions.[95] Whereas injection drug use is uncommon in sub-Saharan Africa, unsafe injection practices in the realm of medical care is another common means of transmission. Such practices also expose medical personnel to the risk of HCV infection.[96] Vertical transmission is low but is more significant in the setting of coinfection with HIV.[97]

Europe

The WHO estimated prevalence of HCV in Europe is 1%.[81] In 2006, the European Center for Disease Control and Prevention (ECDC) estimated the overall incidence of newly reported HCV cases to be 6.7 cases per 100,000 inhabitants, with the highest rates reported in Ireland (29.1 cases per 100,000), Finland (22.5 cases per 100,000), Sweden (21.8 cases per 100,000), and the United Kingdom (17.2 cases per 100,000). Although reporting procedures varied from country to country[98] and direct comparisons are difficult to perform, the overall trend of incidence from 1995 to 2005 was increasing.[11] Males (64.4%) were more commonly infected than females (35.6%), and more than half of the hepatitis C cases (53%) were reported in the age group 25 to 44 years.[98] In Northern Europe, the overall prevalence was 0.1% to 1%, affecting adults aged 30 to 50 years the most. In Central Europe, the HCV prevalence is intermediate, ranging from 0.2% in the Netherlands to 1.2% in France. In Southern Europe including Spain, Italy, Greece, and Southern France, the overall prevalence ranges from 2.5% to 3.5%, with isolated areas in Italy and Greece having higher prevalence rates of 7% to 20% of the general population. In these countries, iatrogenic spread that occurred more than 50 years ago led to a high prevalence in the older population, followed 3 decades later by another high prevalence in the younger individuals who practice IVDU.[99] In Northern Italy, HCV prevalence was highest in the native Italians older than 75 years.[56]

The predominant means of transmission in the past was by blood transfusion, but improved blood supply safety over the past 15 to 20 years has paved the way for IVDU to become the main route for HCV transmission. The expansion of IVDU practices to Western Europe is accompanied by an even more dramatic increase in

Eastern Europe. Despite advances in the safety of medical procedures, nosocomial infections continue to occur even in developed countries. Finally, immigration from endemic areas contributes to the increased prevalence of HCV in Europe. In the Netherlands, immigrants accounted for 56% of prevalent HCV infection. In Spain, immigrants from Latin America had a lower rate of HCV at 0.9%, but immigrants from sub-Saharan Africa, Asia, and Pakistan had a much higher rate of 9% to 11%.[99]

Eastern Mediterranean

The WHO estimated prevalence of HCV in the Eastern Mediterranean region is 4.6% or 21.3 million [81] This region includes Egypt, the largest reservoir of HCV in the world with its prevalence rate of 11% to 14% or 8 to 10 million inhabitants, of whom 5 to 7 million have active viremia.[100,101] The major source of infection is exposure to intravenous tartar emetic that was used to control schistosomiasis 20 to 50 years ago.[102] The rate of infection is lowest in Cairo and Alexandria at 8%, intermediate in rural areas along the Nile south of Cairo (Middle and Upper Egypt) at 8% to 16%, and highest in rural areas of Nile Delta or Lower Egypt, at 15%.[101] The infection is more common in males and in older individuals.[103] The large reservoir of HCV among the older Egyptians allowed for efficient transmission via infected blood products and medical equipment.[101] Hepatitis C is the cause of most cases of HCC (60% to 78.5%) in this country.[46,104] Of note, more than 90% of HCV infections are due to genotype 4.[87,105]

Another country with high endemicity for HCV is Pakistan. The Pakistan Medical Research Council estimate the prevalence of HCV at 4.9% or 8.8 million people.[49] The prevalence of the disease has increased since 2005, when the Prime Minister Program for Prevention and Control of Hepatitis started to provide free treatment to poor patients on a limited scale, and more people underwent testing and sought treatment. The pattern of transmission in Pakistan is not well documented, but parenteral exposure to infected needles and blood are believed to be important risk factors. In addition, community barber shops where infected razors can transmit the infection are another route. IVDU and sexual transmission are minor contributors in HCV transmission in this country.[106]

South-East Asia

The WHO South-East Asia region has an estimated HCV prevalence of 2.15% or 32.3 million individuals.[81] Availability of data on member states is limited, but a summary of published reports as well as on WHO estimates was presented in 1999 (**Table 1**), with the exception of Timor-Leste, which had not yet gained its independence from Indonesia at that time.

India is the most populated country in this region, but data on the prevalence of HCV in the general population is scant. Whereas HCV prevalence is estimated at 1.5% to 4.3% in voluntary blood donors,[107,108] a few population-based studies reported a prevalence of 0.71% to 2.02%.[108] On the other hand, HCV prevalence is even more significantly higher in commercial blood donors at 55.3% to 87.3%.[109,110] In the most systematic population-based study performed in West Bengal involving 10,737 inhabitants from 9 villages, the HCV infection was directly proportional to the age, with the highest prevalence in the age group older than 60 years and the lowest in the age group younger than 10 years. No gender difference was observed.[111] Hepatitis C is incriminated as the cause of liver cirrhosis in 3.3% to 31.5% of cases and of HCC in 15.1% to 42% of cases.[112] The major source of transmission is transfusion of blood and blood products, although the rate has been decreasing since the mandatory screening for HCV in blood donors has been introduced as late as 2002 in some areas.[113] IVDU is a significant problem in north-east India and the rest of the

Table 1
Hepatitis C prevalence in the WHO South-East Asia Region, 1999

Country	Prevalence Rate (%)	Prevalence Rate (in Million Inhabitants)
Bangladesh	2.4	3.08
Bhutan	1.3	0.03
India	1.2	12.08
Indonesia	2.5	5.31
Maldives	1.8	0.005
Myanmar	3.9	1.92
Nepal	1.1	0.26
DPR Korea	1.6	0.38
Sri Lanka	1.4	0.26
Thailand	2.9	1.75

country, and in the only study that addressed the prevalence of HCV in this population, an alarming 92% was reported in 77 intravenous drug users from Manipur Saha. Hemodialysis is another risk factor, with prevalence rates of 4.3% to 28% being observed in dialyzed patients. Health care workers, particularly dentists, are also at higher risk.[108]

In Thailand, the prevalence of HCV antibody is 1.37% to 2.9% in voluntary blood donors,[114,115] with a 2:1 ratio amongst males to females.[115] Intravenous drug use is the most common route of transmission, followed by previous blood or blood product transfusion, sharing of razors, and unsafe injection practices.[116] The prevalence is as high as 86% to 92.5% in the IVDU populations,[117,118] while commercial sex workers also have a prevalence rate of 9.5%.[119]

In Indonesia, the prevalence of HCV is 2.1% in blood donors, in whom prior blood transfusion, IVDU, surgery, and acupuncture were identified as risk factors.[120] In Myanmar, 2.5% of the 363 healthy subjects were found to be positive for HCV in 2002.[121]

Western Pacific

The WHO Western Pacific region has an estimated HCV prevalence of 3.9% or 62.2 million people.[81] Due to the high endemicity of HBV in this region, fewer data are available on HCV. About 3.2% of China's population, or 38 million individuals, were found to have HCV in a national epidemiologic survey done in 1992 to 1995. The most important means of transmission is IVDU, and the HCV incidence in the intravenous drug user cohort is as high as 3.6 cases per 100 person-years.[122] The pooled HCV infection rate among the IVDU population throughout the country was 61.4%, with the risk increasing with duration of IVDU as well as with HIV coinfection.[123]

In Japan, the estimated HCV prevalence is 2% or 2 million people.[124] The prevalence is directly proportional to age, with the highest rate of 7% seen in individuals older than 70 years.[125] The modes of transmission include blood transfusions, IVDU, and unsafe needle use in medical practice before 1980. Hepatitis C is the major etiological factor for HCC in Japan, where HBV is not endemic.[126]

In Australia, the estimated HCV prevalence was 210,000 at the end of 2001, and the estimated incidence of new HCV infection was higher at 16,000 in 2001 compared with 11,000 in 1997.[127] About 80% to 90% of HCV infections are attributed to IVDU, and the increasing prevalence is attributed to the increasing prevalence of this practice despite the introduction of needle and syringe programs in the late 1980s.[128] In contrast, Samoa and American Samoa have a low HCV prevalence, estimated at 0.2% to 0.6% of the population, which is reflective of the low rate of IVDU as well as unsafe medical practices in these countries.[129]

SUMMARY

The global epidemiology of hepatitis B and C continues to evolve, mostly toward a decline in the prevalence of the disease. Improvement in the control of hepatitis B has been largely achieved with implementation of a more global HBV vaccine program. The most recent available data from 2001 indicate that 126 (66%) of 191 WHO member states had universal infant or childhood HBV vaccination programs. In the 6 WHO regions, the proportion of children younger than 1 year who were vaccinated fully was 65% in the Western Pacific region, 58% in the Americas region, 45% in the European region, 41% in the Eastern Mediterranean region, 9% in the South-East Asian region, and 6% in the African region. Overall, an estimated 32% of children younger than 1 year were vaccinated fully with the 3-dose hepatitis B vaccination series worldwide. Although significant progress has been made, there still is a large void to be filled in the global prevention of HBV transmission.[130]

The transmission of HCV has been greatly impacted by mandatory screening of blood donors in most countries in the world. However, IVDU continues to be a major source of infection, and the practice may be on the rise in several areas. Continuing public education regarding the risks of exposure to infected paraphernalia as well as household items such as razors is necessary. To date, there is no effective vaccine available for HCV, which greatly limits the ability to prevent the disease from the grass roots. The efficacy of antiviral therapy for HCV, although steadily escalating, still has a large room for improvement. Treatment of HCV is also costly and access to the medications is limited, particularly in underdeveloped countries. Efforts need to be continued to address these public health issues that afflict many parts of the world.

REFERENCES

1. WHO. Global immunization data. 2009. Available at: http://www.who.int/ immunization/newsroom/GID_english.pdf. Accessed February 1, 2009.
2. Perz JF, Armstrong GL, Farrington LA, et al. The contributions of hepatitis B virus and hepatitis C virus infections to cirrhosis and primary liver cancer worldwide. J Hepatol 2006;45(4):529–38.
3. WHO. Hepatitis B vaccines. Wkly Epidemiol Rec 2004;79(28):253–64.
4. CDC. Epidemiology and prevention of vaccine-preventable diseases (The pink book). 10th edition. Waldorf (MD): Public Health Foundation; 2008.
5. Schaefer S. Hepatitis B virus genotypes in Europe. Hepatol Res 2007;37(S1): S20–6.
6. Devesa M, Pujol FH. Hepatitis B virus genetic diversity in Latin America. Virus Res 2007;127(2):177–84.
7. Lai CL, Ratziu V, Yuen MF, et al. Viral hepatitis B. Lancet 2003;362(9401): 2089–94.
8. Wai CT, Fontana RJ. Clinical significance of hepatitis B virus genotypes, variants, and mutants. Clin Liver Dis 2004;8(2):321–52, vi.
9. Fung SK, Lok AS. Hepatitis B virus genotypes: do they play a role in the outcome of HBV infection? Hepatology 2004;40(4):790–2.
10. Schaefer S. Hepatitis B virus taxonomy and hepatitis B virus genotypes. World J Gastroenterol 2005;13:14–21.

11. Rantala M, van de Laar MJW. Surveillance and epidemiology of hepatitis B and C in Europe—a review. Euro Surveill 2008;13(4–6):1–8.
12. Schaefer S. Hepatitis B virus: significance of genotypes. J Viral Hepat 2005; 12(2):111–24.
13. Kao JH. Hepatitis B viral genotypes: clinical relevance and molecular characteristics. J Gastroenterol Hepatol 2002;17(6):643–50.
14. Glynn SA, Kleinman SH, Schreiber GB, et al. Trends in incidence and prevalence of major transfusion-transmissible viral infections in US blood donors, 1991 to 1996. Retrovirus Epidemiology Donor Study (REDS). JAMA 2000; 284(2):229–35.
15. US CDC. Disease burden from hepatitis A, B and C. Available at: http://www.cdc.gov/Hepatitis/Statistics.htm#section1. Accessed March 9, 2009.
16. McMahon BJ, Schoenberg S, Bulkow L, et al. Seroprevalence of hepatitis B viral markers in 52,000 Alaska Natives. Am J Epidemiol 1993;138(7):544–9.
17. Smith N, Yusuf H, Averhoff F. Surveillance and prevention of hepatitis B virus transmission. Am J Public Health 1999;89(1):11–3.
18. Euler GL, Wooten KG, Baughman AL, et al. Hepatitis B surface antigen prevalence among pregnant women in urban areas: implications for testing, reporting, and preventing perinatal transmission. Pediatrics 2003;111(5 Part 2):1192–7.
19. Public Health Agency of Canada. Hepatitis B factsheet. Available at: http://www.phac-aspc.gc.ca/hcai-iamss/bbp-pts/hepatitis/hep_b-eng.php. Accessed March 3, 2009.
20. Public Health Agency of Canada. Canadian immunization guide, 7th edition, 2006. Available at: http://www.phac-aspc.gc.ca/publicat/cig-gci/p04-hepb-eng.php. Accessed March 3, 2009.
21. Zhang J, Zou S, Giulivi A. Epidemiology of hepatitis B in Canada. Can J Infect Dis 2001;12(6):345–50.
22. Custer B, Sullivan SD, Hazlet TK, et al. Global epidemiology of hepatitis B virus. J Clin Gastroenterol 2004;38(10 Suppl 3):S158–68.
23. Silveira TR, da Fonseca JC, Rivera L, et al. Hepatitis B seroprevalence in Latin America. Rev Panam Salud Publica 1999;6(6):378–83.
24. Tanaka J. Hepatitis B epidemiology in Latin America. Vaccine 2000;18(Suppl 1): S17–9.
25. Fay OH. Hepatitis B in Latin America: epidemiologic patterns and eradication strategy. The Latin American Regional Study Group. Vaccine 1990;8(Suppl):86–92.
26. Torres J. Hepatitis B and hepatitis delta virus infection in South America. Gut 1996;38(Suppl 2):S48–55.
27. Gish RG, Gadano AC. Chronic hepatitis B: current epidemiology in the Americas and implications for management. J Viral Hepat 2006;13(12):787–98.
28. Torres JR, Machado IV. Special aspects of hepatitis B virus and delta virus infection in Latin America. Infect Dis Clin North Am 1994;8(1):13–27.
29. Torres JR, Mondolfi A. Protracted outbreak of severe delta hepatitis: experience in an isolated Amerindian population of the Upper Orinoco basin. Rev Infect Dis 1991;13(1):52–5.
30. Kiire C. Hepatitis B infection in sub-Saharan Africa: the African regional Study Group. Vaccine 1990;8:107–12.
31. Parkin DM, Bray FI, Devesa SS. Cancer burden in the year 2000. The global picture. Eur J Cancer 2001;37(Suppl 8):S4–66.
32. Kirk GD, Lesi OA, Mendy M, et al. The gambia liver cancer study: infection with hepatitis B and C and the risk of hepatocellular carcinoma in West Africa. Hepatology 2004;39(1):211–9.

33. Kew MC. Progress towards the comprehensive control of hepatitis B in Africa: a view from South Africa. Gut 1996;38(Suppl 2):S31-6.
34. Sall Diallo A, Sarr M, Fall Y, et al. [Hepatitis B infection in infantile population of Senegal]. Dakar Med 2004;49(2):136-42 [in French].
35. Coursaget P, Leboulleux D, Yvonnet B, et al. Hepatitis B virus infection and hepatocellular carcinoma in Senegal: prevalence and prevention. J Gastroenterol Hepatol 1993;8:s128-33.
36. Roingeard P, Diouf A, Sankale JL, et al. Perinatal transmission of hepatitis B virus in Senegal, West Africa. Viral Immunol 1993;6(1):65-73.
37. Marinier E, Barrois V, Larouze B, et al. Lack of perinatal transmission of hepatitis B virus infection in Senegal, West Africa. J Pediatr 1985;106(5):843-9.
38. Whittle H, Inskip H, Bradley AK, et al. The pattern of childhood hepatitis B infection in two Gambian villages. J Infect Dis 1990;161(6):1112-5.
39. Kiire C. The epidemiology and control of hepatitis B in sub-Saharan Africa. Prog Med Virol 1993;40:141-56.
40. Pawlotsky JM, Belec L, Gresenguet G, et al. High prevalence of hepatitis B, C, and E markers in young sexually active adults from the Central African Republic. J Med Virol 1995;46(3):269-72.
41. Edmunds WJ, Medley GF, Nokes DJ, et al. Epidemiological patterns of hepatitis B virus (HBV) in highly endemic areas. Epidemiol Infect 1996;117(2):313-25.
42. Akani CI, Ojule AC, Opurum HC, et al. Sero-prevalence of hepatitis B surface antigen (HBsAg) in pregnant women in Port Harcourt, Nigeria. Niger Postgrad Med J 2005;12(4):266-70.
43. Oshitani H, Kasolo FC, Mpabalwani M, et al. Prevalence of hepatitis B antigens in human immunodeficiency virus type 1 seropositive and seronegative pregnant women in Zambia. Trans R Soc Trop Med Hyg 1996;90(3):235-6.
44. Viviani S, Carrieri P, Bah E, et al. 20 years into the Gambia Hepatitis Intervention Study: assessment of initial hypotheses and prospects for evaluation of protective effectiveness against liver cancer. Cancer Epidemiol Biomarkers Prev 2008;17(11):3216-23.
45. Tsebe KV, Burnett RJ, Hlungwani NP, et al. The first five years of universal hepatitis B vaccination in South Africa: evidence for elimination of HBsAg carriage in under 5-year-olds. Vaccine 2001;19(28-29):3919-26.
46. Lehman EM, Wilson ML. Epidemiology of hepatitis viruses among hepatocellular carcinoma cases and healthy people in Egypt: a systematic review and meta-analysis. Int J Cancer 2009;124(3):690-7.
47. Sherif MM, Abou-Aita BA, Abou-Elew MH, et al. Hepatitis B virus infection in upper and lower Egypt. J Med Virol 1985;15(2):129-35.
48. Beasley RP. Hepatitis B virus. The major etiology of hepatocellular carcinoma. Cancer 1988;61(10):1942-56.
49. 9M suffering from hepatitis C, Senate told, in The News International. Islamabad, 2009. Available at: http://www.thenews.com.pk/print1.asp?id=166167. Accessed March 8, 2009.
50. Khattak MF, Salamat N, Bhatti FA, et al. Seroprevalence of hepatitis B, C and HIV in blood donors in northern Pakistan. J Pak Med Assoc 2002;52(9): 398-402.
51. Butt T, Amin MS. Seroprevalence of hepatitis B and C infections among young adult males in Pakistan. East Mediterr Health J 2008;14(4):791-7.
52. Alizadeh AH, Ranjbar M, Ansari S, et al. Seroprevalence of hepatitis B in Nahavand, Islamic Republic of Iran. East Mediterr Health J 2006;12(5): 528-37.

53. Goudeau A. Epidemiology and eradication strategy for hepatitis B in Europe. The European Regional Study Group. Vaccine 1990;8(Suppl):S113–6 [discussion: S134–8].

54. ECDC. Hepatitis B: epidemiological situation. Available at: http://www.ecdc. europa.eu/en/Health_Topics/hepatitis/hepatitisB/aer_07.aspx. Accessed March 4, 2009.

55. WHO regional office for Europe, hepatitis B, 2007. Available at: http://data.euro. who.int/cisid/?TabID=197787. Accessed March 4, 2009.

56. Fabris P, Baldo V, Baldovin T, et al. Changing epidemiology of HCV and HBV infections in Northern Italy: a survey in the general population. J Clin Gastroenterol 2008;42(5):527–32.

57. Veldhuijzen IK, Smits LJ, van de Laar MJ. The importance of imported infections in maintaining hepatitis B in The Netherlands. Epidemiol Infect 2005;133(1): 113–9.

58. Linglof TO. Hepatitis B in parts of former USSR. Scand J Infect Dis 1995;27(3): 299–300.

59. Magdzik WW. Hepatitis B epidemiology in Poland, Central and Eastern Europe and the newly independent states. Vaccine 2000;18(Suppl 1):S13–6.

60. Adamo B, Stroffolini T, Sagliocca L, et al. Ad hoc survey of hepatitis B vaccination campaign in newborns of HBsAg positive mothers and in 12-year-old subjects in southern Italy. Vaccine 1998;16(8):775–7.

61. Mele A, Tancredi F, Romano L, et al. Effectiveness of hepatitis B vaccination in babies born to hepatitis B surface antigen-positive mothers in Italy. J Infect Dis 2001;184(7):905–8.

62. Stroffolini T, Mele A, Tosti ME, et al. The impact of the hepatitis B mass immunisation campaign on the incidence and risk factors of acute hepatitis B in Italy. J Hepatol 2000;33(6):980–5.

63. Tanprasert S, Somjitta S. Trend study on HbsAg prevalence in Thai voluntary blood donors. Southeast Asian J Trop Med Public Health 1993;24(Suppl 1):S43–5.

64. Chub-uppakarn S, Panichart P, Theamboonlers A, et al. Impact of the hepatitis B mass vaccination program in the southern part of Thailand. Southeast Asian J Trop Med Public Health 1998;29(3):464–8.

65. Luksamijarulkul P, Thammata N, Tiloklurs M. Seroprevalence of hepatitis B, hepatitis C and human immunodeficiency virus among blood donors, Phitsanulok Regional Blood Center, Thailand. Southeast Asian J Trop Med Public Health 2002;33(2):272–9.

66. Luksamijarulkul P, Watagulsin P, Sujirarat D. Hepatitis B virus seroprevalence and risk assessment among personnel of a governmental hospital in Bangkok. Southeast Asian J Trop Med Public Health 2001;32(3):459–65.

67. Pramoolsinsap C, Pukrittayakamee S, Desakorn V. Hepatitis B problem in Thailand. Southeast Asian J Trop Med Public Health 1986;17(2):219–28.

68. Tandon BN, Acharya SK, Tandon A. Epidemiology of hepatitis B virus infection in India. Gut 1996;38(Suppl 2):S56–9.

69. WHO regional office for South-East Asia, India. Core program clusters. Family and community health. Hepatitis B. Available at: http://www.whoindia.org/EN/Section6/Section8_26.htm#a4. Accessed March 6, 2009.

70. WHO regional office for South-East Asia. Prevention of hepatitis B in India, New Delhi, August 2002. Available at: http://whqlibdoc.who.int/searo/2002/SEA_Hepat.-5. pdf. Accessed March 6, 2009.

71. John TJ, Abraham P. Hepatitis B in India: a review of disease epidemiology. Indian Pediatr 2001;38(11):1318–25.

72. Chowdhury A, Santra A, Chaudhuri S, et al. Prevalence of hepatitis B infection in the general population: a rural community based study. Trop Gastroenterol 1999;20(2):75–7.
73. Gust ID. Epidemiology of hepatitis B infection in the Western Pacific and South East Asia. Gut 1996;38(Suppl 2):S18–23.
74. Lingao AL, Domingo EO, West S, et al. Seroepidemiology of hepatitis B virus in the Philippines. Am J Epidemiol 1986;123(3):473–80.
75. Lansang MA. Epidemiology and control of hepatitis B infection: a perspective from the Philippines, Asia. Gut 1996;38(Suppl 2):S43–7.
76. Lin HH, Kao JH, Chang TC, et al. Secular trend of age-specific prevalence of hepatitis B surface and e antigenemia in pregnant women in Taiwan. J Med Virol 2003;69(4):466–70.
77. Yao GB. Importance of perinatal versus horizontal transmission of hepatitis B virus infection in China. Gut 1996;38(Suppl 2):S39–42.
78. Chang MH, Chen CJ, Lai MS, et al. Universal hepatitis B vaccination in Taiwan and the incidence of hepatocellular carcinoma in children. Taiwan childhood hepatoma study group. N Engl J Med 1997;336(26):1855–9.
79. Huang K, Lin S. Nationwide vaccination: a success story in Taiwan. Vaccine 2000;18(Suppl 1):S35–8.
80. Recommendations for prevention and control of hepatitis C virus (HCV) infection and HCV related chronic disease. MMWR Recomm Rep 1998;47(RR-19):1–39.
81. WHO. Hepatitis C, WHO fact sheet no. 164, revised 2000. Available at: http://www.who.int/mediacentre/factsheets/fs164/en/. Accessed March 8, 2009.
82. Alter MJ. Epidemiology of hepatitis C virus infection. World J Gastroenterol 2007;13(17):2436–41.
83. Houghton M. Hepatitis C viruses. In: Fields BN, Knipe DM, Howley PM, editors. Fields virology. 3rd edition. Philadelphia: Lippincott-Raven; 1996. p. 1036–58.
84. Mondelli MU, Silini E. Clinical significance of hepatitis C virus genotypes. J Hepatol 1999;31(Suppl 1):65–70.
85. Global surveillance and control of hepatitis C. Report of a WHO consultation organized in collaboration with the Viral Hepatitis Prevention Board, Antwerp, Belgium. J Viral Hepat 1999;6(1):35–47.
86. Nguyen MH, Keeffe EB. Chronic hepatitis C: genotypes 4 to 9. Clin Liver Dis 2005;9(3):411–26, vi.
87. Kamal SM, Nasser IA. Hepatitis C genotype 4: what we know and what we don't yet know. Hepatology 2008;47(4):1371–83.
88. Armstrong GL, Wasley A, Simard EP, et al. The prevalence of hepatitis C virus infection in the United States, 1999 through 2002. Ann Intern Med 2006; 144(10):705–14.
89. Public Health Agency of Canada. Evaluation of the hepatitis C prevention, support and research program 1999/2000-2005/2006. Available at: http://www.phac-aspc.gc.ca/publicat/2008/er-re-hepc/er-re-hepc1-eng.php#ref. Accessed March 9, 2009.
90. Gully PR, Tepper ML. Hepatitis C. CMAJ 1997;156(10):1427–30.
91. Ono-Nita SK, Nita ME, Carrilho FJ. Hepatitis C: facts in numbers. Arq Gastroenterol 2006;43(2):71–2.
92. Santos-Lopez G, Sosa-Jurado F, Vallejo-Ruiz V, et al. Prevalence of hepatitis C virus in the Mexican population: a systematic review. J Infect 2008;56(4): 281–90.
93. Chiquete E, Panduro A. Low prevalence of anti-hepatitis C virus antibodies in Mexico: a systematic review. Intervirology 2007;50(1):1–8.

94. Madhava V, Burgess C, Drucker E. Epidemiology of chronic hepatitis C virus infection in sub-Saharan Africa. Lancet Infect Dis 2002;2(5):293–302.
95. Jeannel D, Fretz C, Traore Y, et al. Evidence for high genetic diversity and long-term endemicity of hepatitis C virus genotypes 1 and 2 in West Africa. J Med Virol 1998;55(2):92–7.
96. Simonsen L, Kane A, Lloyd J, et al. Unsafe injections in the developing world and transmission of bloodborne pathogens: a review. Bull World Health Organ 1999;77(10):789–800.
97. Gibb DM, Goodall RL, Dunn DT, et al. Mother-to-child transmission of hepatitis C virus: evidence for preventable peripartum transmission. Lancet 2000; 356(9233):904–7.
98. ECDC. Annual epidemiological report on communicable diseases in Europe 2008. Available at: http://ecdc.europa.eu/en/files/pdf/Publications/081215_AER_long_2008.pdf. Accessed March 4, 2009.
99. Esteban JI, Sauleda S, Quer J. The changing epidemiology of hepatitis C virus infection in Europe. J Hepatol 2008;48(1):148–62.
100. Strickland GT, Elhefni H, Salman T, et al. Role of hepatitis C infection in chronic liver disease in Egypt. Am J Trop Med Hyg 2002;67(4):436–42.
101. Strickland GT. Liver disease in Egypt: hepatitis C superseded schistosomiasis as a result of iatrogenic and biological factors. Hepatology 2006;43(5):915–22.
102. Frank C, Mohamed MK, Strickland GT, et al. The role of parenteral antischisto-somal therapy in the spread of hepatitis C virus in Egypt. Lancet 2000; 355(9207):887–91.
103. Nafeh MA, Medhat A, Shehata M, et al. Hepatitis C in a community in Upper Egypt: I. Cross-sectional survey. Am J Trop Med Hyg 2000;63(5–6):236–41.
104. Raza SA, Clifford GM, Franceschi S. Worldwide variation in the relative importance of hepatitis B and hepatitis C viruses in hepatocellular carcinoma: a systematic review. Br J Cancer 2007;96(7):1127–34.
105. Ramia S, Eid-Fares J. Distribution of hepatitis C virus genotypes in the Middle East. Int J Infect Dis 2006;10(4):272–7.
106. Raja NS, Janjua KA. Epidemiology of hepatitis C virus infection in Pakistan. J Microbiol Immunol Infect 2008;41(1):4–8.
107. Khaja MN, Munpally SK, Hussain MM, et al. Hepatitis C virus: the Indian scenario. Curr Sci 2002;83(3):219–24.
108. Mukhopadhya A. HCV: the Indian scenario. Trop Gastroenterol 2006;27(3):105–10.
109. Jha J, Banerjee K, Arankalle VA. A high prevalence of antibodies to hepatitis C virus among commercial plasma donors from Western India. J Viral Hepat 1995; 2(5):257–60.
110. Nandi J, Bhawalkar V, Mody H, et al. Detection of HIV-1, HBV and HCV antibodies in blood donors from Surat, western India. Vox Sang 1994;67(4):406–7.
111. Chowdhury A, Santra A, Chaudhuri S, et al. Hepatitis C virus infection in the general population: a community-based study in West Bengal, India. Hepatology 2003;37(4):802–9.
112. WHO Regional Office for South-East Asia. Blood safety and clinical technology. Policy guidelines on HCV testing report of an informal consultation, New Delhi, 21-22nd December, 1999. Available at: http://www.searo.who.int/en/Section10/Section17/Section58/Section220_217.htm. Accessed March 11, 2009.
113. Hazra SC, Chatterjee S, Das Gupta S, et al. Changing scenario of transfusion-related viral infections. J Assoc Physicians India 2002;50:879–81.
114. Wiwanitkit V. Anti HCV seroprevalence among the voluntary blood donors in Thailand. Hematology 2005;10(5):431–3.

115. Luksamijarulkul P, Thammata N, Sujirarat D, et al. Hepatitis C virus infection among Thai blood donors: antibody prevalence, risk factors and development of risk screening form. Southeast Asian J Trop Med Public Health 2004;35(1): 147–54.

116. Tanwandee T, Piratvisuth T, Phornphutkul K, et al. Risk factors of hepatitis C virus infection in blood donors in Thailand: a multicenter case-control study. J Med Assoc Thai 2006;89(Suppl 5):S79–83.

117. Jittiwutikarn J, Thongsawat S, Suriyanon V, et al. Hepatitis C infection among drug users in northern Thailand. Am J Trop Med Hyg 2006;74(6):1111–6.

118. Hansurabhanon T, Jiraphongsa C, Tunsakun P, et al. Infection with hepatitis C virus among intravenous-drug users: prevalence, genotypes and risk-factor-associated behaviour patterns in Thailand. Ann Trop Med Parasitol 2002; 96(6):615–25.

119. Luksamijarulkul P, Deangbubpha A. Hepatitis C antibody prevalence and risk factors of some female sex workers in Thailand. Southeast Asian J Trop Med Public Health 1997;28(3):507–12.

120. Sulaiman HA, Julitasari, Sie A, et al. Prevalence of hepatitis B and C viruses in healthy Indonesian blood donors. Trans R Soc Trop Med Hyg 1995;89(2): 167–70.

121. Kyi KP, Aye M, Oo KM, et al. Population and patients with liver ailments in Myanmar. Reg Health Forum 2002;6(1):1–6. Available at: http://www.searo. who.int/EN/Section1243/Section1310/Section1343/Section1344/Section1355_ 5302.htm. Accessed March 11, 2009.

122. Garten RJ, Lai S, Zhang J, et al. Rapid transmission of hepatitis C virus among young injecting heroin users in Southern China. Int J Epidemiol 2004;33(1): 182–8.

123. Xia X, Luo J, Bai J, et al. Epidemiology of hepatitis C virus infection among injection drug users in China: systematic review and meta-analysis. Public Health 2008;122(10):990–1003.

124. Higuchi M, Tanaka E, Kiyosawa K. Epidemiology and clinical aspects on hepatitis C. Jpn J Infect Dis 2002;55(3):69–77.

125. Yoshizawa H. Hepatocellular carcinoma associated with hepatitis C virus infection in Japan: projection to other countries in the foreseeable future. Oncology 2002;62(Suppl 1):8–17.

126. Iino S. Relationship between infection with hepatitis C virus and hepatocellular carcinoma in Japan. Antivir Ther 1998;3(Suppl 3):143–6.

127. Law MG, Dore GJ, Bath N, et al. Modelling hepatitis C virus incidence, prevalence and long-term sequelae in Australia, 2001. Int J Epidemiol 2003;32(5): 717–24.

128. Dore GJ, Law M, MacDonald M, et al. Epidemiology of hepatitis C virus infection in Australia. J Clin Virol 2003;26(2):171–84.

129. Armstrong GL, Williams IT, Maga UA, et al. Hepatitis C virus infection in Samoa and American Samoa. Am J Trop Med Hyg 2006;74(2):261–2.

130. Gacic-Dobo M, Mayers G, Birmingham M, et al. Global progress toward universal childhood hepatitis B vaccination, 2003. MMWR Morb Mortal Wkly Rep 2003;52(36):868–70.

Occupational Exposure of Health Care Personnel to Hepatitis B and Hepatitis C: Prevention and Surveillance Strategies

Taranisia MacCannell, MSc, PhD[a],*, Angela K. Laramie, MPH[b],
Ahmed Gomaa, MD, ScD, MSPH[c], Joseph F. Perz, DrPH, MA[a]

KEYWORDS

- Hepatitis B • Hepatitis C • Occupational exposure
- Bloodborne pathogens

Health care personnel represent a vital workforce that aims to preserve and improve the health of others. Among the 35 million health care personnel employed worldwide, percutaneous injuries have been estimated to result in approximately 16,000 hepatitis C and 66,000 hepatitis B virus infections annually.[1] Within the United States, an estimated 14.4 million workers are employed in the health care industry, with more than 5.7 million employed in hospitals alone.[2] The landscape of health care delivery is changing, and increases in staff workload and patient complexity may have an impact on the likelihood of occupational injuries. Ensuring health care personnel safety is a challenge that must be met with multifaceted approaches to prevention.

The findings and conclusions of this article are those of the authors and do not necessarily represent the official position of the Centers for Disease Control and Prevention.
[a] Division of Healthcare Quality Promotion, Centers for Disease Control and Prevention, 1600 Clifton Road NE, MS-A31, Atlanta, GA 30333, USA
[b] Sharps Injury Surveillance Project, Occupational Health Surveillance Program, Massachusetts Department of Public Health, 250 Washington Street, 6th Floor, Boston, MA 02108, USA
[c] Division of Surveillance Hazard Evaluation and Health Studies, National Institute for Occupational Safety and Health, Centers for Disease Control and Prevention, CINC Building HAMIL Room B 301, MS R17, Cincinnati, OH 45226, USA
* Corresponding author.
E-mail address: tmaccannell@cdc.gov (T. MacCannell).

In the context of health care–associated occupational bloodborne pathogen risks, the US Public Health Service (USPHS) defines health care personnel as persons (eg, employees, students, contractors, attending clinicians, public safety workers, or volunteers) whose activities involve contact with patients or with blood or other body fluids from patients in a health care, laboratory, or public safety setting.[3] Injuries involving needles and other sharps in health care are associated with the transmission of many pathogens, but the pathogens of most immediate concern during patient care activities are hepatitis B virus (HBV), hepatitis C virus (HCV), and HIV.[4–6] These infections are associated with chronic disease and significant morbidity and mortality.

The majority of exposures to bloodborne pathogens in health care personnel are preventable.[4,7] Protection from bloodborne pathogen exposures is fundamental to health care personnel and patient safety. The prevention of sharps injuries is an important aspect of eliminating the transmission of bloodborne pathogens to health care personnel, and contributes to establishing safe workplace environments. This review describes the epidemiology of HBV and HCV in health care personnel, with a focus on current prevention and postexposure management strategies and provides examples of surveillance programs used to monitor and manage these exposures.

RISK OF HEPATITIS B AND HEPATITIS C VIRUS EXPOSURES IN HEALTH CARE PERSONNEL

The probability of acute HBV or HCV infection after the exposure to a susceptible person depends on the route of exposure, the concentration of infectious virions in body fluids, the volume of infective material transferred, and the immune status of the recipient.[8] HBV is primarily transmitted by percutaneous and mucosal exposure to blood and body fluids. Risk of contracting HBV depends on the degree of exposure to infectious fluids and the presence of hepatitis B surface antigen, anti–hepatitis B core antibody, or hepatitis B e antigen, the latter being a marker for increased viral replication and infectivity. Positive hepatitis B e antigen status is indicative of high viral titers (eg, $10^7–10^9$ virions/mL).[9,10] The highest titers of HBV are found in blood and, as such, contribute to the increased risk of transmission from sharps injuries. Other body fluids are not as conducive to the transmission of HBV.[3]

HBV can persist in the environment for prolonged periods and can remain infective in dried blood at room temperature for more than a week.[8,11] Transmission of HBV may also occur in health care settings through exposures to nonintact skin from contaminated environmental surfaces or equipment that has been inadequately cleaned and disinfected.[8] Infective concentrations of HBV have been detected on environmental surfaces in the absence of visible blood. Its ability to remain stable outside the human host supports other evidence that HBV infection may occur through direct and indirect means of transmission.[3] HCV in dried blood samples has been shown to remain infective for 16 hours.[12] Environmental exposures to HCV in health care settings seem to have a limited role in the transmission of HCV and likely pose a low risk. HBV and HCV are enveloped viruses and are sensitive to the appropriate Environmental Protection Agency–registered disinfectants and sterilants, and when employed correctly can be an effective measure to reduce environmental contamination.[13]

The risk of HBV seroconversion after a percutaneous injury ranges from 23% to 62% in unvaccinated persons and is dependent on the hepatitis B e antigen status of the source.[8] Surveys performed in the 1990s of unvaccinated US health care personnel showed that serologic evidence of past or current HBV infection was present in approximately 22% of respondents, a figure typically three to five times greater than in the US general population. Among respondents, surgeons reported the highest HBV seroprevalence of 28% among unvaccinated personnel.[14–16] Survey data from the 1990s suggest that 13% of surgeons have evidence for current or past HBV infection, but 64% also received the HBV vaccine.[17] The estimated number of HBV infections in health care personnel has decreased from greater than 10,000 in 1983 to fewer than 400 in 2002 after the integration of routine HBV immunization through facility-based occupational health and safety policies, USPHS guidelines, and regional Occupational Safety and Health Administration (OSHA) mandates.[3,18,19] The seroprevalence of HBV in health care personnel is now fivefold less than in the US population (approximately 4%).[7,16,19]

HCV transmission is most efficient after percutaneous injury, with deep punctures or extensive blood exposures enhancing the likelihood of transmission.[20–22] It is unclear whether mucosal or nonintact skin exposures have a significant role in transmission, as these are rarely documented transmission events.[3,23] The risk of infection was elevated 11-fold when the HCV load of a positive source patient was greater than 10^6 virions/mL compared with patients with viral loads less than 10^4 virions/mL.[21] Approximately 50 to 150 cases of HCV transmission in health care personnel are conservatively estimated to occur each year in the United States.[24] The seropreva-lence of HCV in US health care providers is approximately 0.5% to 2.0%, which is comparable to that in the general population.[14,25–28] From the available evidence, these data hold true even among provider groups that are at greater risk for expo-sures, such as surgical or dialysis staff.[16,29,30]

Overall, the risk of HCV transmission after percutaneous exposure is low, approxi-mately 1.8%.[3] In contrast to the infrequent occurrence of chronic HBV infection in newly infected adults (5%–10%), chronic infection occurs in the majority (70%–85%) of persons with newly acquired HCV infection.[25,31,32] Avoidance of exposures and adherence to Standard Precautions and engineering and work practice controls remain essential to preventing occupational infection, given that no vaccination or postexposure prophylaxis measures are currently available for HCV.

Epidemiology of Sharps Injuries in Health Care Personnel

Despite increasing implementation of strategies to prevent injuries and blood expo-sures, more than 385,000 needlestick injuries were estimated to occur annually in US hospitals during 1997 to 1998.[26] In addition, the burden of exposures in nonhos-pital settings is ill defined. Other estimates, which considered under-reporting and nonhospital care, projected that the overall magnitude of sharps injuries in US health care could approach 600,000 to 800,000 per year.[27,28,33] These projections may have improved in light of the Needlestick Safety and Prevention Act, which passed in 2000.

Needlestick injuries can occur during a broad spectrum of health care activities if appropriate engineering and work practice controls or a supportive culture of safety are not present. Data from the National Surveillance System for Healthcare Workers (NaSH) indicates that the largest proportions of injuries occurred in patient rooms (35%) and operating theaters (28%). Hollow-bore needlestick injuries, which are asso-ciated with exposures to greater volumes of blood and increased transmission risks, occurred more frequently than solid sharps injuries (54% vs 40%).[7,34] The Centers for Disease Control and Prevention (CDC) estimates that at least 56% of percutaneous injuries involving hollow-bore needles are preventable.[35] Data from NaSH summa-rizing 30,945 reported exposures from 1995 to 2007 showed that 12.6% of source patients were infected with HBV (1.4%), HCV (8.4%), or HIV (4.5%); 1.7% were co-infected with HCV and HIV.[7] Among nurses and physicians, approximately 25% of reported hollow-bore sharps injuries were deemed to have been preventable by the use of safer devices.[36] Almost two-thirds of all reported injuries occurred with devices without safety features. Among the 3316 injuries involving sharps devices that were equipped with safety features, 23% involved a failure to activate the safety feature and 41% involved an injury that occurred before the safety component was meant to be activated.[7]

Risk Groups for Exposure

According to NaSH, 82% of blood and body fluid exposures were from percutaneous injuries, with the largest proportions of exposures reported in nurses (41%) and physicians (30%). Nursing staff generally outnumber other health care professionals who provide direct patient care and represent the occupational group most affected by percutaneous injuries, a reflection of their close and repeated contacts with patients.[35,37–39]

Although all health care staff who provide direct patient contact are at-risk for exposure to blood and body fluids, surgical and obstetrics staff are often cited as a particularly vulnerable occupational group.[40–43] NaSH data have shown that 28% of injuries were reported in operating theaters.[7] In other studies examining the risk of injury in operating theaters, 93% of injuries were sharps related, and in half of those injuries, suture needles were implicated.[43,44] According to one study from the 1990s, percutaneous injuries were reported in 7% to 10% of all gynecologic surgeries.[17] In a survey of medical students, 30% of reported needlesticks occurred frequently in operating theaters.[45] An increased likelihood of percutaneous injuries are associated with surgeries that take longer than 6 hours, surgeries with patient blood losses greater than 1000 mL, and many personnel crowding the surgical field.[44]

PROTECTING HEALTH CARE PERSONNEL FROM EXPOSURE TO BLOOD AND BODY FLUIDS
Measures to Prevent Exposures (Primary Prevention)

Prevention of blood and body fluid exposures represents a cornerstone of occupational programs in health care. The OSHA Bloodborne Pathogens Standard issued in 1991 established provisions to minimize bloodborne exposures to health care personnel.[46,47] The Standard focused on adherence to universal precautions (subsequently incorporated into Standard Precautions), which was intended as the standard of care for all patients in all health care facilities, regardless of their known or suspected infectious status.[48,49] Precautions include measures to protect health care personnel and patients from exposures to blood and body fluids. Other key provisions of the OSHA Bloodborne Pathogens Standard require employers to provide hepatitis B vaccine to staff, involve staff in the selection of safer needle devices, develop an exposure control plan and postexposure protocols, and provide engineering and work practice controls, personal protective equipment, and annual training. The Standard was revised and expanded by the Needlestick Safety and Prevention Act of 2000, which explicitly mandated the use of engineered safety devices to eliminate the risk of sharps injuries.[48] The updated Standard also requires employers to maintain a log of injuries from contaminated sharps.[47]

Vaccination

Hepatitis B vaccine became available in 1982, and in that same year was recommended for US health care personnel by the Advisory Committee on Immunization Practices.[50] Three intramuscular doses of hepatitis B vaccine induce a protective antibody response in more than 90% of healthy recipients.[2,31] Adults who develop a protective antibody response are protected from clinical disease and chronic infection. The duration of vaccine protection is under investigation, but available evidence indicates that nearly all vaccinated persons who respond have lifelong immunity against HBV infection.[31] Health care personnel who do not respond to the primary vaccine series should receive a second three-dose series; non-responders should be evaluated for chronic infection.[3] Booster doses of hepatitis B vaccine are not necessary, and periodic serologic testing to monitor antibody concentrations after completion of the vaccine series is not recommended.[3]

Adherence to the Advisory Committee on Immunization Practices guidelines was bolstered by the 1991 OSHA Bloodborne Pathogens Standard where employers were required to provide hepatitis B vaccination at no cost, and resulted in increased coverage levels in US health care personnel. For example, 51% of health care personnel were vaccinated for hepatitis B in 1992. This figure rose to 67% in 1995. As of 2003, it was estimated that 75% of health care personnel were vaccinated for HBV, with the highest coverage levels among staff physicians and nurses.[51-53] Since US recommendations for hepatitis B vaccination of infants and children were published in 1991, more than 90% coverage of children with the complete HBV immunization series has been achieved. Universal infant immunization with hepatitis B vaccine is expected to lead to increased levels of HBV immunity in persons now entering the health care workforce.[54-56]

There is currently no vaccine to prevent HCV infection. Instead, efforts continue to focus on prevention activities, such as adherence to Standard Precautions, safe work practices, counseling, and education for health care personnel.[8]

Hierarchy of Controls

A concept widely promoted in industrial hygiene, the "hierarchy of controls" principle, has been applied to bloodborne pathogen exposure prevention by providing structure and priority setting for key interventions. The hierarchy establishes priorities for hazard reductions in the workplace. The first priority is the elimination or reduction of sharps use. Examples of this strategy include switching, to the extent possible, to needleless intravenous delivery systems; oral, noninjectable medications; and glues or other adhesives in place of traditional sutures.[57-59]

If a potential hazard cannot be removed, the next priority is to mitigate the hazard through the use of engineering controls. Examples of this second strategy include making sharps disposal containers accessible at their point of use and using engineered safety devices.[60,61] Such devices can have active or passive safety mechanisms to prevent sharps injury; devices requiring activation typically require users to engage the safety feature after use whereas more passive devices operate by self-sheathing, self-blunting, or automatically retracting after use.[4]

The federal OSHA standard and several state-based regulations have required that devices with engineered sharps injury prevention features must be provided by employers. When applied correctly, safety devices have had dramatic effects on the rates of injury to health care personnel.[39,62,63] For example, increased uptake of safety-engineered devices reduced the incidence of percutaneous injuries from 34/1000 full-time equivalents to 14/1000 full-time equivalents after their implementation in one hospital.[64] Activities that had the most significant impact from the switch to safer devices were catheter insertion procedures, with nursing staff reporting the largest reduction in injuries.[64]

When sharps elimination and engineering control strategies are not available or are insufficient, the use of work practice controls and personal protective equipment represents important adjunct prevention activities. Work practice controls are often used during surgical and obstetric procedures when the use of exposed sharps cannot be avoided. In operating rooms, these controls include using instruments to grasp needles, retract tissue, and unload/load needles and scalpels; giving verbal announcements when passing sharps; using a basin or neutral zone to avoid hand-to-hand passing of sharps; opting for noninvasive procedures when possible (eg, endoscopy, laser, or electrocautery procedures); and using round-tipped scalpel blades and blunt suture needles.[65] In surgical settings, the practice of double gloving can significantly reduce the volume of blood exposure from sharps injuries compared with wearing single gloves.[4,66–72] To support the effective implementation of the hierarchy of controls for sharps injury prevention, comprehensive training on the use of safety-engineered devices, work practice controls, and personal protective equipment are essential.[36]

Standard Precautions

Standard Precautions are a series of recommended practices that establish the standard of care for all patients in health care. It encompasses the principles of Universal Precautions and body substance isolation that were introduced by the CDC in the 1980s after the emergence of HIV/AIDS. Standard Precautions are based on the possibility that all blood, body fluids, secretions, excretions (except sweat), nonintact skin, and mucous membranes may contain transmissible infectious agents, such as HBV and HCV.[49] The application of Standard Precautions during patient care is determined by the nature of the anticipated exposure to blood or body fluids. Hand hygiene is a critical component within Standard Precautions as an effective practice to reduce the risk of exposures to blood and body fluids and patient-to-patient transmission of bacterial and non-bloodborne viral pathogens. Personal protective equipment consists of the use of gowns; disposable gloves; and masks, face shields, or goggles for patient care when there is potential for contact with blood and body fluids. Safe injection practices were made explicit within Standard Precautions in the 2007 Guideline for Isolation Precautions: Preventing Transmission of Infectious Agents in Healthcare Settings; these recommendations were intended to clarify appropriate needle, syringe, and medication handling to prevent patient-to-patient, health care provider-to-patient, and patient-to-health care provider transmission of HBV, HCV, and other pathogens.[49]

Education and Training

In the United States, OSHA requirements mandate yearly training on the prevention of blood and body fluid exposures. Training in and responsibility for basic infection control is increasingly emphasized by accrediting and regulatory agencies, such as the Joint Commission and the Center for Medicare and Medicaid Services. The need for education was illustrated by a survey of physicians and nurses in the United Kingdom, where only 50% of nurses and 32% of physicians correctly identified the risks of acquiring HBV after a sharps injury.[73] Similarly, only 35% of nurses and 44% of physicians could correctly identify HCV transmission risks. Among this cohort, 28% of physicians did not report their needlestick injuries despite being a specialty most likely to sustain sharps injuries. NaSH data echoed these results with an estimated 30% of percutaneous injury events likely to be reported by surgeons, whereas 53% of physicians and nurses were likely to report their injuries.[7] Barriers to reporting exposures cited by personnel included lack of time and a perception of minimal risk.[32] Deficiencies in staff training and education on basic injection safety and risk assessment are associated with personnel underestimating the risk of HBV and HCV transmission, even when a patient source was known to be HBV or HCV positive.[74–78] The availability and promotion of regular training for staff is a low-cost measure that can improve adherence to Standard Precautions to safe work practices to prevent injuries and exposures.[48]

Culture of Safety in the Workplace

Maintaining a culture of safety is a shared responsibility. Management and staff should collectively work to encourage and promote safety in the workplace. Every member within an organization is accountable for the safety of patients and the work environment. Development of and adherence to policies for reporting injuries and mechanisms for identifying and resolving injury hazards are important parts of this commitment. Successful safety cultures in the workplace are also contingent on every individual being accountable for safety and serving as a role model for safer work practices.[4,79] Evidence suggests that organizations that support and promote safety in the workplace may experience overall improvements in infection prevention, including reductions in occupational exposure to bloodborne pathogens. One study demonstrated that facilities with policies to discourage needle recapping practices were likely to have employed needleless intravenous systems, had infection control and safety management personnel available, had routine education on Standard Precautions, and had provisions to encourage personal protective equipment use.[48]

Regulations and Policies

Most health care workers in the United States are protected by the OSHA Bloodborne Pathogens Standard, which outlines measures that employers must take to prevent exposures in workers. As directed by Needlestick Safety and Prevention Act of 2000, OSHA issued a revision in 2001 to the original 1991 Bloodborne Pathogens Standard.[47]

More than 20 states have regulations aimed at sharps injury prevention and surveillance, often extending protections to public sector workers. California was the first state to legislate the use of engineered sharps devices as a revision to the Bloodborne Pathogens Standard in 1998.[60] State OSHA plans, the Center for Medicare and Medicaid Service, and the Joint Commission all have requirements addressing the risk of exposure among health care personnel. The CDC has provided guidelines for the management of occupational exposure to HBV, HCV, and HIV.[3,80] These regulations and guidelines have facilitated the increase in the number of health care personnel who have been vaccinated against HBV, promoted the use of devices with engineered sharps injury prevention features, and improved the provision of appropriate follow-up and treatment for injured or exposed health care personnel.

MEASURES TO PREVENT HEPATITIS B OR HEPATITIS C INFECTION AFTER AN EXPOSURE

Occupational exposures to blood and body fluids should be managed in accordance with established recommendations and guidelines (discussed previously). Health care institutions must have a written policy regarding postexposure case management that includes protocols for obtaining source patient consent to test for HIV, HBV, and HCV. Employees should be provided with information regarding the types of incidents to report, details of how to report incidents, and locations where medical evaluations, counseling, and follow-up are available. Trained personnel should always be available to a facility for postexposure management and follow-up.

Postexposure prophylaxis for HBV requires the evaluation of several factors, such as the hepatitis B surface antigen status of the source and the vaccination and HBV immunity status of the exposed health care worker. After any exposure, unvaccinated health care personnel are recommended to start the hepatitis B vaccination series. If HBV immune globulin is indicated, it should be given as soon as possible, preferably within 24 hours; the effectiveness of HBV immune globulin after 7 days post exposure is unknown (see 2001 USPHS guidelines for detailed recommendations).[3]

Currently, there is no postexposure prophylaxis available for HCV. Health care personnel who are exposed to a confirmed HCV antibody-positive (or unknown status) source should have baseline testing completed for anti-HCV and alanine aminotransferase activity.[3] These tests should be repeated in 4 to 6 months in asymptomatic health care personnel, and any positive anti-HCV should be confirmed with additional molecular diagnostics. Early detection strategies, which call for more frequent and aggressive testing to monitor exposed individuals, have been advocated; USPHS guidelines also indicate that testing for HCV RNA may be performed 4 to 6 weeks after exposure if earlier detection of infection is desired.[3,81,82] In those instances when infection is detected, antiviral therapy may be most effective if it is initiated in the early stages of infection. HCV treatment decisions are complex and underscore the need for appropriate medical referrals and counseling as part of postexposure management.

SURVEILLANCE

Data gathered from surveillance systems have provided valuable information regarding the circumstances surrounding blood exposure incidents and the occupations at risk of such exposures. In turn, this information has proved valuable in guiding prevention efforts. Several platforms for the collection of data on bloodborne pathogen exposures in health care workers are available. National data on sharps injuries in US health care personnel have primarily been reported through the CDC's NaSH and through the Exposure Prevention Information Network (EPINet), based at the International Healthcare Worker Safety Center (**Box 1**). EPINet began data collection in 1992 and currently collects similar data from a network of approximately 33 facilities concentrated in several geographic areas around the country.[28]

NaSH compiled data from 1995 to 2007 with 64 participating hospitals at its peak in 2000. A total of 81 health care facilities contributed data over 12 years of voluntary surveillance, resulting in more than 30,000 reports of blood and body fluid exposures.[7] The NaSH system and user support were discontinued in December 2007 to focus on

---

Box 1
Supplemental resources: tools and guidance for prevention of occupational exposures to bloodborne pathogens

CDC. Division of Healthcare Quality Promotion: http://www.cdc.gov/ncidod/dhqp/index.html

CDC. Division of Viral Hepatitis: http://www.cdc.gov/hepatitis/

CDC. National Institute for Occupational Safety and Health: http://www.cdc.gov/niosh/topics/bbp

CDC. Division of Healthcare Quality Promotion. Workbook for Designing, Implementing, and Evaluating a Sharps Injury Prevention Program: http://www.cdc.gov/sharpssafety

CDC. National Healthcare Safety Network: http://www.cdc.gov/nhsn/hps_bbf.html

International Healthcare Worker Safety Center. The Exposure Prevention Information Network: http://www.healthsystem.virginia.edu/Internet/epinet/

OSHA. Bloodborne pathogens and needlestick prevention: http://www.osha.gov/SLTC/bloodbornepathogens/index.html

U.S. Department of Veterans Affairs. Needle safety: http://www1.va.gov/vasafety/page.cfm?pg=119

Commonwealth of Massachusetts, Office of Health and Human Services, Department of Public Health. Occupational Health Surveillance Program, Sharps Injury Surveillance and Prevention Project: http://www.mass.gov/dph/ohsp

the development of the Healthcare Personnel Safety Component of the CDC National Healthcare Safety Network (NHSN) and no longer accepted data as of January 2008.

Several states conduct sharps injury surveillance, although some are limited to public sector workers or the private sector. Although most of these are voluntary systems, Massachusetts hospitals licensed by the Department of Public Health report to the Department of Public Health sharps injuries among health care personnel. This surveillance system has captured data from all licensed hospitals since 2002, and as of 2008, there were more than 23,000 recorded percutaneous injuries among health care personnel in 99 licensed hospitals (Massachusetts Department of Public Health. Massachusetts Sharps Injury Surveillance and Prevention Project. Boston: Occupational Health Surveillance Program, unpublished data, 2009).

NHSN incorporates aspects of NaSH in a new Healthcare Personnel Safety Component was launched in August 2009 for facility enrollment and data collection. The Blood and Body Fluids Exposure Module will collect data on exposure events, risk factors, and devices causing injury; health care worker demographics; details on exposure follow-up and required prophylaxis; and relevant laboratory results. Participating facilities will have the option of collecting details on longitudinal exposure management. This module integrates many features from the NaSH system but offers increased functionality, technical support, and access to real-time data and reporting. The Blood and Body Fluids Exposure Module will allow users to calculate rates of exposure, and seroconversion, and assist in the management of injuries and allow facilities to track injuries within their facility and compare injury rates against aggregated NHSN data.

SUMMARY

Prevention strategies to eliminate occupational exposures to HBV and HCV in health care have a growing evidence base to support their adoption. In the United States, dramatic reductions in HBV infection in health care personnel followed successful efforts to vaccinate health care personnel. Further efforts to increase vaccination coverage and monitor the long-term effectiveness of hepatitis B immunization are warranted. Collectively, the use of Standard Precautions, engineering controls, and other workplace strategies can substantially reduce or even eliminate the risk of percutaneous and mucous membrane exposures to HBV and HCV. Surveillance systems (eg, NHSN and EPINet) to track and monitor trends of blood and body fluid exposures are useful for improving understanding of the circumstances that contribute to occupational exposures to HBV and HCV and for developing solutions—technologic or educational—to close the gap on preventable exposures.

Further research is needed to better define the impact of knowledge, attitudes, and current practices in at-risk health care personnel on their risk of bloodborne pathogen exposures. With the availability and wider implementation of engineering controls, such as sharps with safety features, there is a need to evaluate their efficacy as a component for prevention but also explore the challenges to their appropriate implementation. In summary, exposure to infectious blood and body fluids represents an important occupational hazard for health care providers. A comprehensive approach to HBV and HCV prevention is needed in all health care settings to assure basic worker and patient protections (see **Box 1**).

REFERENCES

1. Pruss-Ustun A, Rapiti E, Hutin Y. Estimation of the global burden of disease attributable to contaminated sharps injuries among health-care workers. Am J Ind Med 2005;48(6):482–90.

2. US Department of Labor. Bureau of Labor Statistics (BLS) current population survey. Table 18, 2006. Available at: http://www.bls.gov/cps/cpsaat18.pdf. Accessed April, 2009.

3. Centers for Disease Control and Prevention. Updated U.S. Public Health Service guidelines for the management of occupational exposures to HBV, HCV, and HIV and recommendations for postexposure prophylaxis. MMWR Recomm Rep 2001; 50(RR-11):1–52.

4. Centers for Disease Control and Prevention. Sharps injury prevention: workbook for designing, implementing, and evaluating a sharps injury prevention program. Atlanta (GA): Centers for Disease Control and Prevention; 2008. Available at: http://www.cdc.gov/sharpssafety. Accessed February, 2009.

5. Sepkowitz KA. Occupationally acquired infections in health care workers. Part II. Ann Intern Med 1996;125(11):917–28.

6. Perry J, Jagger J, Parker G. Nurses and needlesticks, then and now. Nursing 2003;33(4):22.

7. Centers for Disease Control and Prevention. The National Surveillance System for Healthcare Workers—blood and body fluid exposures summary report, June 1995-December 2007. Atlanta (GA): Centers for Disease Control and Prevention; unpublished data.

8. Beltrami EM, Perz JF. Occupational exposures to bloodborne pathogens. In: Carrico R, editor. Text for infection control and epidemiology. 3rd edition. Washington, DC: Association for Professionals in Infection Control; 2009.

9. Alter HJ, Seeff LB, Kaplan PM, et al. Type B hepatitis: the infectivity of blood positive for e antigen and DNA polymerase after accidental needlestick exposure. N Engl J Med 1976;295(17):909–13.

10. Shikata T, Karasawa T, Abe K, et al. Hepatitis B e antigen and infectivity of hepatitis B virus. J Infect Dis 1977;136(4):571–6.

11. Bond WW, Favero MS, Petersen NJ, et al. Survival of hepatitis B virus after drying and storage for one week. Lancet 1981;1(8219):550–1.

12. Kamili S, Krawczynski K, McCaustland K, et al. Infectivity of hepatitis C virus in plasma after drying and storing at room temperature. Infect Control Hosp Epidemiol 2007;28(5):519–24.

13. Sattar SA, Tetro J, Springthorpe VS, et al. Preventing the spread of hepatitis B and C viruses: where are germicides relevant? Am J Infect Control 2001;29(3):187–97.

14. Gerberding JL. Incidence and prevalence of human immunodeficiency virus, hepatitis B virus, hepatitis C virus, and cytomegalovirus among health care personnel at risk for blood exposure: final report from a longitudinal study. J Infect Dis 1994;170(6):1410–7.

15. Lanphear BP. Trends and patterns in the transmission of bloodborne pathogens to health care workers. Epidemiol Rev 1994;16(2):437–50.

16. Beltrami EM, Williams IT, Shapiro CN, et al. Risk and management of blood-borne infections in health care workers. Clin Microbiol Rev 2000;13(3):385–407.

17. Short LJ, Bell DM. Risk of occupational infection with blood-borne pathogens in operating and delivery room settings. Am J Infect Control 1993;21(6):343–50.

18. Williams IT, Perz JF, Bell BP. Viral hepatitis transmission in ambulatory health care settings. Clin Infect Dis 2004;38(11):1592–8.

19. Mahoney FJ, Stewart K, Hu H, et al. Progress toward the elimination of hepatitis B virus transmission among health care workers in the United States. Arch Intern Med 1997;157(22):2601–5.

20. Puro V, Petrosillo N, Ippolito G, et al. Hepatitis C virus infection in healthcare workers. Infect Control Hosp Epidemiol 1995;16(6):324–6.

21. Yazdanpanah Y, De Carli G, Migueres B, et al. Risk factors for hepatitis C virus transmission to health care workers after occupational exposure: a European case-control study. Clin Infect Dis 2005;41(10):1423–30.

22. De Carli G, Puro V, Ippolito G. Risk of hepatitis C virus transmission following percutaneous exposure in healthcare workers. Infection 2003;31(Suppl 2):22–7.

23. Beltrami EM, Kozak A, Williams IT, et al. Transmission of HIV and hepatitis C virus from a nursing home patient to a health care worker. Am J Infect Control 2003; 31(3):168–75.

24. Sepkowitz KA, Eisenberg L. Occupational deaths among healthcare workers. Emerg Infect Dis 2005;11(7):1003–8.

25. Centers for Disease Control and Prevention. Recommendations for prevention and control of hepatitis C virus (HCV) infection and HCV-related chronic disease. Centers for Disease Control and Prevention. MMWR Recomm Rep 1998; 47(RR-19):1–39.

26. Panlilio AL, Orelien JG, Srivastava PU, et al. Estimate of the annual number of percutaneous injuries among hospital-based healthcare workers in the United States, 1997–1998. Infect Control Hosp Epidemiol 2004;25(7):556–62.

27. Henry K, Campbell S. Needlestick/sharps injuries and HIV exposure among health care workers. National estimates based on a survey of U.S. hospitals. Minn Med 1995;78(11):41–4.

28. EPINet. Exposure prevention information network data reports. University of Virginia: International Healthcare Worker Safety Center, 1999. Available at: http://www.healthsystem.virginia.edu/Internet/epinet/. Accessed April, 2009.

29. Zuckerman AJ. Occupational exposure to hepatitis B virus and human immuno-deficiency virus: a comparative risk analysis. Am J Infect Control 1995;23(5): 286–9.

30. Struve J, Aronsson B, Frenning B, et al. Prevalence of antibodies against hepatitis C virus infection among health care workers in Stockholm. Scand J Gastroenterol 1994;29(4):360–2.

31. Centers for Disease Control and Prevention. A comprehensive immunization strategy to eliminate transmission of hepatitis B virus infection in the United States. Recommendations of the Advisory Committee on Immunization Practices (ACIP) part II: immunization of adults. MMWR Morb Mortal Wkly Rep 2006;55(16):1–25.

32. Tandberg D, Stewart K, Doezma D. Under-reporting of contaminated needlestick injuries in emergency healthcare workers. Ann Emerg Med 1991;20(1):66–70.

33. Leigh JP, Gillen M, Franks P, et al. Costs of needlestick injuries and subsequent hepatitis and HIV infection. Curr Med Res Opin 2007;23(9):2093–105.

34. Cardo DM, Bell DM. Bloodborne pathogen transmission in health care workers. Risks and prevention strategies. Infect Dis Clin North Am 1997;11(2):331–46.

35. McCormick RD, Mcisch MG, Ircink FG, et al. Epidemiology of hospital sharps injuries: a 14-year prospective study in the pre-AIDS and AIDS eras. Am J Med 1991;91(3B):301S–7S.

36. Castella A, Vallino A, Argentero PA, et al. Preventability of percutaneous injuries in healthcare workers: a year-long survey in Italy. J Hosp Infect 2003;55(4):290–4.

37. Mansour AM. Needlestick injury in the OR: facts and prevention. J Ophthalmic Nurs Technol 1989;8(6):222–4.

38. Ruben FL, Norden CW, Rockwell K, et al. Epidemiology of accidental needle-puncture wounds in hospital workers. Am J Med Sci 1983;286(1):26–30.

39. Whitby M, McLaws ML, Slater K. Needlestick injuries in a major teaching hospital: the worthwhile effect of hospital-wide replacement of conventional hollow-bore needles. Am J Infect Control 2008;36(3):180–6.

40. Doebbeling BN, Vaughn TE, McCoy KD, et al. Percutaneous injury, blood exposure, and adherence to standard precautions: are hospital-based health care providers still at risk? Clin Infect Dis 2003;37(8):1006–13.

41. Babcock HM, Fraser V. Differences in percutaneous injury patterns in a multi-hospital system. Infect Control Hosp Epidemiol 2003;24(10):731–6.

42. Dement JM, Epling C, Ostbye T, et al. Blood and body fluid exposure risks among health care workers: results from the duke health and safety surveillance system. Am J Ind Med 2004;46(6):637–48.

43. Bakaeen F, Awad S, Albo D, et al. Epidemiology of exposure to blood borne pathogens on a surgical service. Am J Surg 2006;192(5):e18–21.

44. Myers DJ, Epling C, Dement J, et al. Risk of sharp device-related blood and body fluid exposure in operating rooms. Infect Control Hosp Epidemiol 2008;29(12): 1139–48.

45. Patterson JM, Novak CB, Mackinnon SE, et al. Needlestick injuries among medical students. Am J Infect Control 2003;31(4):226–30.

46. Occupational exposure to bloodborne pathogens—OSHA. Final rule. Fed Regist 1991;56(235):64004–182.

47. Occupational exposure to bloodborne pathogens; needlestick and other sharps injuries; final rule. Occupational Safety and Health Administration (OSHA), Department of Labor. Final rule; request for comment on the information collection (paperwork) requirements. Fed Regist 2001;66(12):5318–25.

48. Vaughn TE, McCoy KD, Beekmann SE, et al. Factors promoting consistent adherence to safe needle precautions among hospital workers. Infect Control Hosp Epidemiol 2004;25(7):548–55.

49. Siegel JD, Rhinehart E, Jackson M, et al. 2007 guideline for isolation precautions: preventing transmission of infectious agents in healthcare settings. June 2007.

50. Centers for Disease Control and Prevention. Recommendation of the Immunization Practices Advisory Committee (ACIP) inactivated hepatitis B virus vaccine. MMWR Morb Mortal Wkly Rep 1982;31(24):317–22, 327–8.

51. Agerton TB, Mahoney FJ, Polish LB, et al. Impact of the bloodborne pathogens standard on vaccination of healthcare workers with hepatitis B vaccine. Infect Control Hosp Epidemiol 1995;16(5):287–91.

52. Simard EP, Miller JT, George PA, et al. Hepatitis B vaccination coverage levels among healthcare workers in the United States, 2002–2003. Infect Control Hosp Epidemiol 2007;28(7):783–90.

53. Averhoff F, Mahoney F, Coleman P, et al. Immunogenicity of hepatitis B vaccines. Implications for persons at occupational risk of hepatitis B virus infection. Am J Prev Med 1998;15(1):1–8.

54. Centers for Disease Control and Prevention. A comprehensive immunization strategy to eliminate transmission of hepatitis B virus infection in the United States: recommendations of the Advisory Committee on Immunization Practices (ACIP); part 1: immunization of infants, children, and adolescents. MMWR Morb Mortal Wkly Rep 2005;54(RR-16):1–23.

55. Centers for Disease Control and Prevention. National state and urban area vaccination coverage among children aged 19–35 months—United States, 2004. MMWR Morb Mortal Wkly Rep 2005;54(29):717–21.

56. Behrman AJ, Shofer FS, Green-McKenzie J. Trends in bloodborne pathogen exposure and follow-up at an urban teaching hospital: 1987 to 1997. J Occup Environ Med 2001;43(4):370–6.

57. Gartner K. Impact of a needleless intravenous system in a university hospital. Am J Infect Control 1992;20(2):75–9.

58. Skolnick R, LaRocca J, Barba D, et al. Evaluation and implementation of a needle-less intravenous system: making needlesticks a needless problem. Am J Infect Control 1993;21(1):39–41.
59. Yassi A, McGill ML, Khokhar JB. Efficacy and cost-effectiveness of a needleless intravenous access system. Am J Infect Control 1995;23(2):57–64.
60. National Institute for Occupational Safety and Health. Preventing needlestick injuries in health care settings. November, 1999. Available at: http://www.cdc.gov/niosh/docs/2000-108/. Accessed April, 2009.
61. Occupational Safety and Health Administration. Bloodborne pathogens and nee-dlestick prevention: OSHA standards 2001. Available at: http://www.osha.gov/SLTC/bloodbornepathogens/standards.html. Accessed April, 2009.
62. Cullen BL, Genasi F, Symington I, et al. Potential for reported needlestick injury prevention among healthcare workers through safety device usage and improve-ment of guideline adherence: expert panel assessment. J Hosp Infect 2006; 63(4):445–51.
63. Lamontagne F, Abiteboul D, Lolom I, et al. Role of safety-engineered devices in preventing needlestick injuries in 32 French hospitals. Infect Control Hosp Epide-miol 2007;28(1):18–23.
64. Sohn S, Eagan J, Sepkowitz KA, et al. Effect of implementing safety-engineered devices on percutaneous injury epidemiology. Infect Control Hosp Epidemiol 2004;25(7):536–42.
65. Centers for Disease Control and Prevention. Evaluation of blunt suture needles in preventing percutaneous injuries among health-care workers during gynecologic surgical procedures – New York City, March 1993-June 1994. MMWR Morb Mortal Wkly Rep 1997;46(2):25–9.
66. Wittmann A, Kralj N, Kover J, et al. Study of blood contact in simulated surgical needlestick injuries with single or double latex gloving. Infect Control Hosp Epi-demiol 2009;30(1):53–6.
67. Lefebvre DR, Strande LF, Hewitt CW. An enzyme-mediated assay to quantify inoculation volume delivered by suture needlestick injury: two gloves are better than one. J Am Coll Surg 2008;206(1):113–22.
68. Davis MS. Advanced precautions for today's O.R.: the operating room profes-sional's handbook for the prevention of sharps injuries and bloodborne expo-sures. Atlanta (GA): Sweinbinder Publications LLC; 1999.
69. Lewis J, Short L, Howard R, et al. Epidemiology of injuries by needles and other sharp instruments: minimizing sharp injuries in gynecologic and obstetric opera-tions. Surg Clin North Am 1995;75:1105–21.
70. Raahave D, Bremmelgaard A. New operative technique to reduce surgeon's risk of HIV infection. J Hosp Infect 1991;18(Suppl A):177–83.
71. Loudon M, Stonebridge P. Minimizing the risk of penetrating injury to surgical staff in the operating theatre: towards sharp-free surgery. J R Coll Surg Edinb 1998;43:6–8.
72. Gerberding JL. Procedure-specific infection control for preventing intraoperative blood exposures. Am J Infect Control 1993;21(6):364–7.
73. Stein AD, Makarawo TP, Ahmad MF. A survey of doctors' and nurses' knowledge, attitudes and compliance with infection control guidelines in Birmingham teaching hospitals. J Hosp Infect 2003;54(1):68–73.
74. Davanzo E, Frasson C, Morandin M, et al. Occupational blood and body fluid expo-sure of university health care workers. Am J Infect Control 2008;36(10):753–6.
75. Halpern SD, Asch DA, Shaked A, et al. Inadequate hepatitis B vaccination and post-exposure evaluation among transplant surgeons: prevalence, correlates, and implications. Ann Surg 2006;244(2):305–9.

76. Deisenhammer S, Radon K, Nowak D, et al. Needlestick injuries during medical training. J Hosp Infect 2006;63(3):263–7.
77. Jeffe DB, Mutha S, L'Ecuyer PB, et al. Healthcare workers' attitudes and compliance with universal precautions: gender, occupation, and specialty differences. Infect Control Hosp Epidemiol 1997;18(10):710–2.
78. Burke S, Madan I. Contamination incidents among doctors and midwives: reasons for non-reporting and knowledge of risks. Occup Med (Lond) 1997; 47(6):357–60.
79. Rivers DL, Aday LA, Frankowski RF, et al. Predictors of nurses' acceptance of an intravenous catheter safety device. Nurs Res 2003;52(4):249–55.
80. Panlilio AL, Cardo DM, Grohskopf LA, et al. Updated U.S. Public Health Service guidelines for the management of occupational exposures to HIV and recommendations for postexposure prophylaxis. MMWR Recomm Rep 2005;54(RR-9):1–17.
81. Henderson DK. Managing occupational risks for hepatitis C transmission in the health care setting. Clin Microbiol Rev 2003;16(3):546–68.
82. Puro V, De Carli G, Cicalini S, et al. European recommendations for the management of healthcare workers occupationally exposed to hepatitis B virus and hepatitis C virus. Euro Surveill 2005;10(10):260–4.

Molecular Epidemiology of Health Care– Associated Transmission of Hepatitis B and C Viruses

Scott D. Holmberg, MD, MPH

KEYWORDS

- Molecular epidemiology • Hepatitis B • Hepatitis C
- Health care–related transmission

The term "molecular epidemiology" has been ascribed to a host of different activities that involve gene-sequence analysis. Some examples of molecular epidemiology include modeling exercises of phylogenetic trees to reconstruct epidemics[1]; studies of the evolution of hepatitis C virus (HCV)[2]; rates of nucleotide substitution in the hepatitis B virus (HBV) surface (S) gene[3]; variations in the core promoter/pre-core/core region of HBV genotype C from different sources[4]; analysis of HBV surface antigen mutations[5]; molecular clock analyses of the short-term evolution of HCV[6]; and analyses of clades and surface antigen polymorphisms of HBV.[7]

However, for most epidemiologists, infectious disease and liver specialists, molecular epidemiology of viral hepatitis usually refers to studies of gene-sequence homology in HBV or HCV recovered from people in the community or an institution that allows better characterization and assignment of related clusters of infection. Much of this work was initially based on seminal work looking at HIV in patients of an HIV-infected dentist in Florida in the early 1990s.[8] However, it did not take long for others to adopt laboratory and statistical techniques and apply them to the hepatitis viruses.[9–13] Thus, S-gene sequences from HBV-infected persons on several islands in Indonesia were amplified and compared as early

Division of Viral Hepatitis, National Center for HIV, Hepatitis, TB, and STD Prevention, Centers for Disease Control and Prevention, CDC Mailstop G-37; 1600 Clifton Road, Atlanta, GA 30333, USA
E-mail address: sdh1@cdc.gov

Clin Liver Dis 14 (2010) 37–48
doi:10.1016/j.cld.2009.11.008
1089-3261/10/$ – see front matter. Published by Elsevier Inc.

as 1991 (and showed distinct and different sources of infection).[14] Once the genome for HCV had been better characterized by the early 1990s, molecular-epidemiologic investigations of recipients of immunoglobulin in Ireland[15] and of intravenous drug users in rural communities in the United Kingdom[16] followed shortly thereafter.

Most of these early investigations were phylogenetic analyses (ie, of the genotypes and subgenotypes of HCV or HBV) in investigated outbreak subjects, usually in community settings. It is difficult to ascribe the first hepatitis B or C molecular epidemiology performed in the health care setting, although it seems they were probably investigations of transmission between health care workers and patients, in either direction, in the mid 1990s.[17,18]

As techniques and mechanization improved, studies increasingly focused on hypervariable regions (eg, E1- or E2-gene fragment of HCV and the S-gene segment of HBV) as opposed to less variable segments coding genotype (eg, the NS5B region of HCV). Recently, the ability to examine the whole genome may supplant gene-fragment analysis as the standard of viral hepatitis molecular epidemiology (see *Techniques* discussed later).

PROBLEMS AND OBSTACLES IN INVESTIGATING HEPATITIS B VIRUS OR HEPATITIS C VIRUS IN THE HEALTH CARE SETTING

Persons who do not investigate outbreaks may sometimes not appreciate the complexities and difficulties of shoe-leather epidemiology of HBV and HCV in the health care setting. Much hard work goes into detection and delineation of outbreaks before molecular epidemiology can occur; in fact, molecular epidemiology usually confirms what is already suspected from patients and from dogged investigation of a cluster of cases. The usual problems of investigating outbreaks are compounded in the health care setting where professional pride and fear of litigation make respondents less likely than usual to cooperate with investigators.

Thus, before discussing the techniques and utility of molecular epidemiology of HBV and HCV outbreaks in hospitals; clinics; and other settings, such as nursing homes, it is worthwhile to examine the steps and obstacles to regular epidemiology of viral hepatitis in such settings. Each step in the process of detecting and delineating an outbreak has problems and reduces the likelihood of successful molecular epidemiology to confirm the sources of transmission (**Fig. 1**).

Only a minority of acute cases of HBV and HCV infection in the United States associated with a health care source are even detected. The lack of symptoms in most infected persons; the long incubation periods, usually 2 months or more between infection and symptoms, such as jaundice; lack of thorough questioning of persons with incident hepatitis B or hepatitis C; disinclination to believe that health care could be the source of viral-hepatitis infection; inadequate testing; poor charting and record keeping; and many other factors may obscure the association between patients and the hospital or clinic source of infection.

Reporting of hepatitis B and hepatitis C cases to health authorities is spotty. Only 36 states report chronic HCV and only 39 states report chronic HBV through national surveillance to the US Centers for Disease Control and Prevention (CDC). For example, states such as California, with large general and hepatitis-infected populations, do not report; and other states, such as Massachusetts, presently have more than 10-ft high backlogs of cases to enter into their state and national surveillance system. As detection of incident hepatitis C, based on HCV–antibody-positivity plus a high alanine aminotransferase or symptoms, such as jaundice, relies on first

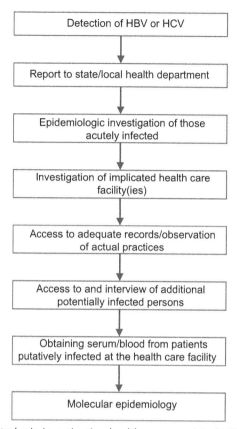

Fig. 1. Steps and obstacles in investigating health care–associated HBV and HCV.

detecting any chronic HCV infection, it is clear that most cases of acute HCV infection are missed by health authorities.

Only some states and city health departments have the manpower and resources to investigate new cases of hepatitis B and hepatitis C, and in those interviews exposure to parenteral drugs or procedures may not even be queried. Occasional transmissions of HBV and HCV in the health care setting, such as from one patient or health care worker (HCW) to only one or two other patients, may easily be missed and are unlikely to be detected at the local or state level. Thus, 25% to 50% of incident hepatitis B and hepatitis C cases reported to the CDC do not have a definition of risk factor or source of infection.[19] Many cases associated with health care transmission are surely never detected by authorities; however, occasionally an alert health department does so.[20]

In the United States, patients may easily refuse to answer or cooperate with a health department investigation of the source of infection (although, fortunately, most do cooperate). However, identifying and interviewing such patients, who may be very sick, have died, have moved, or are otherwise unable to help with an investigation, can often be difficult. Further, only symptomatic patients will be identified for follow-up or investigation.

Implicated health care facilities have a clear motive not to be exposed as having lapses in their infection-control procedures and some will raise procedural, administrative, or legal barriers to health officials who wish to investigate. Records at the facility may be inadequate or confusing, and the staff may change their behavior in the presence of health investigators. Often, investigations can reach a dead end at the facility.

If other potentially infected persons can be identified, the same problems with accessing, interviewing, and obtaining clinical specimens may occur as those initially investigated; such persons may be very sick, have died, have moved, or are otherwise disinclined to cooperate with an investigation for various reasons.

It is clear that only a small minority of health care–associated transmission in the United States results in investigation and obtaining clinical specimens necessary for molecular epidemiology (see **Fig. 1**).

Accordingly, finding almost three dozen outbreaks of detected and implicated hepatitis B and hepatitis C in nonhospital health care settings in the United States from 1998 to 2008[21] clearly indicates a much larger problem. This situation probably occurs to the same extent in other developed countries[22] and certainly in other less-developed countries.

TECHNIQUES OF MOLECULAR EPIDEMIOLOGY OF HEPATITIS C AND B

Molecular epidemiology starts with amplification of genes by polymerase chain reaction (PCR) for DNA viruses like HBV and reverse-transcriptase PCR for RNA viruses like HCV.[23] Generally, nucleic acid is extracted from clinical specimens, usually serum,[24] and the reverse transcription step is performed if the specimen contains HCV. After drying and re-suspension in buffer, primers whose sequences are complementary to sub-genomic segments of the viral genome are used for bracketing the region in which PCR will be performed. A sense primer and an antisense primer are used. Denaturation, primer annealing, and extension are then performed, using a thermostable DNA polymerase, such as *Taq* polymerase. The presence of an amplification product may be subsequently analyzed on an agarose gel stained with ethidium bromide, or in recent years, automated sequencing of PCR products is performed.

An important issue in the molecular epidemiology of hepatitis C virus, especially as spread from one person to another, is which region of the genome to amplify. In general, the highly (or hyper-)variable region (*HVR1*) of the *E1-E2* gene is the most informative region for study, especially if two samples can be obtained soon after the transmission event, before much evolutionary drift can occur.[25] For more distant events, analysis of genes from *NS5b*, the region determining the genotype of HCV, or from a section of *E1* can be analyzed. **Table 1** shows that *NS5b* (for determination of genotype) and *HVR1* analysis were usually performed in outbreak investigations after 2002.

For Hepatitis B, various segments of the genome have been examined: part or all of pre-core, core, surface, and X- or S-gene regions (**Table 2**). No one has systematically studied which of these fragments would be best for molecular epidemiology in the health care setting, but all of them appear to be sufficiently variable enough to allow assignment of identity between any two recovered samples. Some have looked at S-gene variability (or substitution rate) because earlier molecular epidemiology relied on comparison of this gene.[3,50] However, given its relative shortness, the whole HBV genome has been sequenced and compared in some recent investigations,[22] and such analysis may obviate the need for determining which segment would be best amplified and sequenced for purposes of molecular epidemiology.

Finally, analysis of the homology between amplified gene fragments from various persons suspected to be epidemiologically related may be performed by bootstrap analysis,[51] neighbor-joining methods,[52] or both.

Table 1
Molecular epidemiologic studies of hepatitis C virus

Site (Country)[Number]	Transmission in Health Care Settings			
	Number Potentially Exposed/Tested	Number Infected	Genes Sequenced	References
Patient-to-patient				
Hemodialysis (Germany)	224	14	NS5	Zeuzem et al[23]
Hospital (Sweden)	—	3	NS5	Schvarcz et al[26]
Colonoscopy (France)	—	3	NS3	Bronowicki et al[27]
Hemodialysis (Sweden)	103	17	NS5B	Norder et al[28]
Pediatric Oncology (Sweden)	—	10	HVR1	Widell et al[29]
Hematology (Italy)	294	13	HVR1 (E2)	Silini et al[30]
Autodialysis (France)	20	4	HVR1	Halfon et al[31]
Hemodialysis (Spain)	—	6	HVR1 (E1/E2)	González-Candelas[32]
Hospital (US)	24	5	NS5B and HVR1	Krause et al[33]
Organ/tissue (US)	—	9	NS5B and HVR1	Tugwell et al[34]
Hematology/oncology (US)	494	95	NS5B	Macedo de Oliveira et al[35]
Surgery/general anesthesia (Italy)	796	4	NS5B and HVR1 (E2)	Germain et al[36]
Hemodialysis (Tunisia)	395	12	NS5B and HVR1	Hmaïed[37]
Hemodialysis (Brazil)[15]	106	69	NS5B	Carneiro et al[38]
Colonoscopy (US) [2]	—	6	NS5B and HVR1 (E2)	Labus et al[20]
Hemodialysis (Italy)	—	5	NS5B and HVR1 (E2)	Spada et al[39]
CT with contrast (Spain)	—	6	HVR1 (E2)	Pañella et al[40]
Patient to HCW				
Needlestick (Japan)	—	3	HVR1 (E2)	Suzuki et al[17]
Needlestick (Japan)	37	2	HVR1 (E2)	Mizuno et al [41]
Needlestick (Sweden)	—	2	NS5B	Norder et al[28]
HCW to patient				
Immunoglobulin to prevent Rh sensitization	—	2	HVR1 (E1 and E2)	Hohne & Schrier[18]
Surgeon	222	6	HVR1 (E1 and E2)	Esteban et al[42]
Anesthesiologist	348	2	HVR1	Cody et al[43]

Table 2
Molecular epidemiologic studies of hepatitis B virus

	Transmission in Health Care Settings			
Site (Country) [Number]	Number Potentially Exposed/ Tested	Number Infected	Genes Sequenced	References
Patient-to-patient				
Hospital (Israel)	—	5	pre-core, core	Liang et al[10]
Autohemotherapy (UK)	356	30	surface, core	Webster et al[44]
Hospital (Spain)	14	10	complete genome	Bracho et al[45]
Hemodialysis (UK)	—	2	X region, pre-core, core	Ramalingam et al[46]
HCW to Patient				
Surgeon (US)	144	19	core	Harpaz et al[47]
Surgeons (UK) [4]	—	4	X region, core, surface	[48]
Surgeon (Netherlands)	1564	8	S region	Spijkerman et al[49]

HEPATITIS C IN HEALTH CARE SETTINGS

Hepatitis C is highly prevalent even in developed countries, and minor lapses in needle, syringe, or infusion hygiene can easily result in the infection of many. Thus, despite the many obstacles to detection, investigation and reporting of clusters of cases associated with such health care–associated lapses (see **Fig. 1**), numerous outbreaks, verified by molecular analyses, have nonetheless been reported since 1996 (see **Table 1**).[20,26–43] A common theme in most of these patient-to-patient transmissions has been the reuse of a syringe on an HCV-infected patient, leading to contamination of a multiuse vial or solution, in turn resulting in the infection of subsequent patients.[21]

In the two dozen outbreaks delineated in **Table 1**, molecular epidemiology, especially of the *HVR1* of the *E2* and *E1* regions of the HCV genome were essential in implicating transmission in the health care setting. An outbreak we investigated in concert with the Southern Nevada District Health Department (Las Vegas) was illustrative of many important features of HCV investigation by molecular epidemiologic techniques.[20,53]

Initially, three cases over a 6-month period were detected because the local health department was actively tracking and doing preliminary investigations of acute hepatitis C, an unusual acute viral infection in their district (**Fig. 2**).[53] Again, most health districts in the United States are not able or constituted to investigate non-injection drug use incident cases of hepatitis C. Second, the implicated facility, a colonoscopy clinic, neither legally nor administratively blocked a health department investigation, and CDC investigators, observing normal practice, witnessed reuse of syringes in the administration of the intravenous anesthetic (propofol). Clinic records were hard to interpret, but some colonoscopy patients, seen on the same days after patients known to be chronically HCV-infected, were identified, tested, and found to be HCV

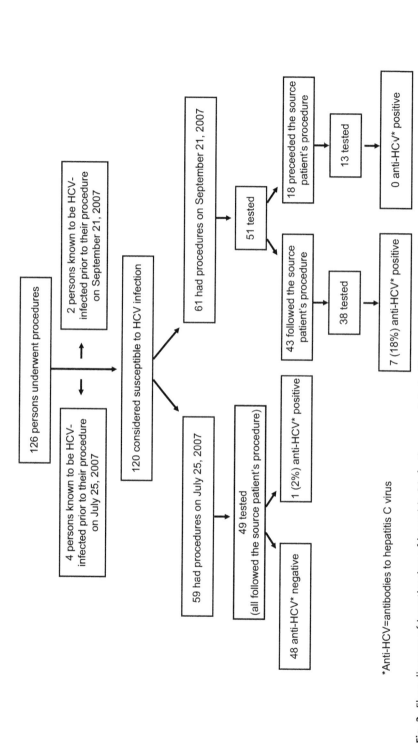

Fig. 2. Flow diagram of investigation of hepatitis C infections associated with procedures at an endoscopy clinic in Las Vegas, Nevada, 2007 to 2008. (*Courtesy of* Gayle E. Fischer, MD, Washington, DC.)

*Anti-HCV=antibodies to hepatitis C virus

The flow diagram contains the following boxes:

- 126 persons underwent procedures
- 4 persons known to be HCV-infected prior to their procedure on July 25, 2007
- 2 persons known to be HCV-infected prior to their procedure on September 21, 2007
- 120 considered susceptible to HCV infection
- 61 had procedures on September 21, 2007
- 59 had procedures on July 25, 2007
- 51 tested
- 49 tested (all followed the source patient's procedure)
- 18 preceeded the source patient's procedure
- 43 followed the source patient's procedure
- 48 anti-HCV* negative
- 1 (2%) anti-HCV* positive
- 13 tested
- 38 tested
- 0 anti-HCV* positive
- 7 (18%) anti-HCV* positive

infected. As the practices associated with infection in this setting, reuse of syringes, pertained for many years, over 60,000 potentially exposed patients seen at the clinic over several years needed to be notified by health authorities to be screened for hepatitis C and other blood borne pathogens (hepatitis B, HIV).

With such widespread testing an additional 77 persons with chronic HCV infection, who denied any other risk than having been seen at the clinic, were identified. However, because of inadequate records and lack of specimens from all other patients seen on many days over a prolonged period (several years), there was no opportunity for molecular epidemiologic matching of specimens from patients newly identified with HCV with other patients seen at the same clinic over that prolonged period; records and patients were no longer available. Although the public health intervention and screening of tens of thousands of potentially exposed patients identified many who did not know they were infected with HCV, these other patients could not be definitely linked to the clinic by molecular epidemiologic means.

Still, molecular techniques used in this epidemic definitively linked many cases to patients who were chronically HCV infected who were seen at this clinic on 2 days in July and September of 2007 (**Fig. 3**). From a public health and policy point of view, molecular epidemiology confirmed the identity of specimens from patients seen at the clinic and added weight and urgency to the public discussion and policies

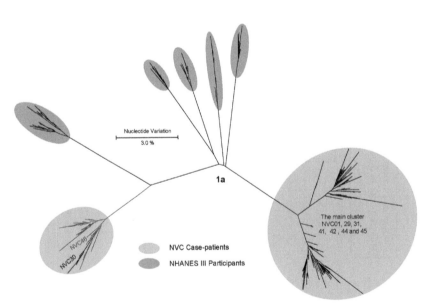

Fig. 3. Highly variable region (HVR)-1 analysis of specimens from an investigation of patients at a colonoscopy clinic in Las Vegas Nevada, 2007 to 2008. A 291–base-pair region within this region (*E1*) was used. Related specimens cluster in genetic relatedness to one another, and in distinction from control specimens collected elsewhere, in patients seen at the clinic on July 25, 2007 (subjects NVC 26 and 30) and on September 21, 2007 (subjects NVC 01, 29, 31, 41, 42, 45, 46). Any two specimens within a cluster have 99.1% or more relatedness. Only unique clonal sequences are shown. NVC, Nevada case (number); NHANES, National Health and Nutrition Survey III, 1988–1994; 1a, HCV genotype 1a. (*Courtesy of* Gayle E. Fischer, MD, Washington, DC.)

on a local and even national level, such as better oversight and inspection of out-of-hospital facilities in Nevada.

HEPATITIS B IN HEALTH CARE SETTINGS

Compared with hepatitis C, far fewer health care–related epidemics have been investigated with molecular techniques (see **Table 2**). The reasons for this are various. In most countries, hepatitis B molecular epidemiology is applied on a national level to look at genotypes, trends, and other factors on a geographic basis.[54,55] In the United States, many acute HBV infections have been acquired in the extended-care setting (assisted-living and nursing-home settings) and have been related to use of shared finger stick devices for blood-glucose monitoring in elderly diabetics.[21,54,56,57] Typically, these transmissions result in a few cases that are infrequently detected and rarely require molecular epidemiology to confirm transmission routes.[21] However, when such hepatitis B outbreaks do occur in the elderly, they are associated with frequent hospitalization and high case fatality,[21] usually 6% or more of those infected. Accordingly, technologic improvements, such as non-parenteral ways of checking blood glucose, and vaccination of susceptible diabetic persons, such as the institutionalized, are being considered as ways to stop this situation.

THE FUTURE OF HEPATITIS MOLECULAR EPIDEMIOLOGY

Genetic techniques have now so supplanted serologic and other manners of typifying organisms that it is fair to state that no modern epidemiologic analysis could afford to forego molecular techniques. The comparatively short length of HCV RNA and HBV DNA, and the rapid adoption of more mechanized and easier gene sequencing, make whole-genome analysis likely to become a standard of molecular epidemiology in the near future. Further, more powerful computer programs are making comparisons of the gene sequences in viral hepatitis from geographically disparate areas easier.

For example, CDC now collects, does whole-genome sequencing, and enters samples of hepatitis A from widely disparate locations in the United States (from the United States/Mexico border to Alaska, to all 48 states in the continental United States) into a computer-data library. DNA sequences from over 200 specimens are now entered, so new hepatitis A can be compared with those previously collected and those collected elsewhere. Eventually, this hepatitis A gene library will give us, as with all molecular epidemiology, better characterization of the immediate sources and causes of outbreaks; a quicker and better epidemiologic understanding of the ultimate source of epidemics (especially food borne) arising elsewhere (eg, another state or country); and insights into the evolution of hepatitis A.

Similar national gene libraries of hepatitis B and C are possible. Although these have traditionally been applied to community-based specimens, there is no reason that similar libraries could not be used to evaluate potential health care–associated specimens. Comparing isolates to such a genetic library would also represent a fundamental shift in health care–associated hepatitis epidemiology, in that investigators would compare specimens from identified patients in the community, rather than trying to track back through health care facility records. Presumably, such a change would allow epidemiologists to more quickly and accurately identify clusters of infections. Although building such a library for HBV and HCV specimens collected nationwide is still far from realized, such a goal is only limited by our imagination and resources.

REFERENCES

1. Ferraro D, Genovese D, Argenti C, et al. Phylogenetic reconstruction of HCV genotype 1b dissemination in a small city centre: the Camporeale model. J Med Virol 2008;80:1723–31.
2. Camp DS, Dimitrova Z, Mitchell RJ, et al. Coordinated evolution of the hepatitis C virus. Proc Natl Acad Sci U S A 2008;105:9685–90.
3. Zaaijer HL, Bouter S, Boot HJ. Substitution rate of the hepatitis B virus surface gene. J Viral Hepat 2008;15:239–45.
4. Truong BX, Yano Y, Seo Y, et al. Variations in the core promoter/pre-core region in HBV genotype C in Japanese and Northern Vietnamese patients. J Med Virol 2007;79:1293–304.
5. Davaalkham D, Ojima T, Uehara R, et al. Analysis of hepatitis B surface antigen mutations in Mongolia: molecular epidemiology and implications for mass vaccination. Arch Virol 2007;152:575–84.
6. Wróbel B, Torres-Puente M, Jiménez N, et al. Analysis of the overdispersed clock in the short-term evolution of hepatitis C virus: using the E1/E2 gene sequences to infer infection dates in a single source outbreak. Mol Biol Evol 2006;23:1242–53.
7. Devesa M, Rodríguez C, León G, et al. Clade analysis and surface antigen polymorphism of hepatitis B virus American genotypes. J Med Virol 2004;72:377–84.
8. Ou CY, Cieselski CA, Myers G, et al. Molecular epidemiology of HIV transmission in a dental practice. Science 1992;256:1155–6.
9. Lin HJ, Lai CL, Lauder IJ, et al. Application of hepatitis B virus (HBV) DNA sequence polymorphisms to the study of HBV transmission. J Infect Dis 1991;164:284–8.
10. Liang TJ, Hasegawa K, Rimon N, et al. A hepatitis B mutant associated with an epidemic of fulminant hepatitis. N Engl J Med 1991;324:1705–9.
11. Pumpens P, Grens E, Nassal M. Molecular epidemiology and immunology of hepatitis B virus infection- an update. Intervirology 2002;45:218–32.
12. Van Belkum A, Niesters HG. Nucleic acid amplification and related techniques in microbiological diagnostics and epidemiology. Cell Mol Biol (Noisy-le-grand) 1995;41:615–23.
13. Norder H, Hammas B, Magnius LO. Typing of hepatitis B virus genomes by a simplified polymerase chain reaction. J Med Virol 1990;31:215–21.
14. Sastrosoewignjo RI, Danjaja B, Okamoto H. Molecular epidemiology of hepatitis B virus in Indonesia. J Gastroenterol Hepatol 1991;6:491–8.
15. Power JP, Lawlor E, Davidson F, et al. Molecular epidemiology of an outbreak of infection with hepatitis C virus in recipients of anti-D immunoglobulin. Lancet 1995;345:1211–3.
16. Majid A, Holmes R, Desselberger U, et al. Molecular epidemiology of hepatitis C virus infection among intravenous drug users in rural communities. J Med Virol 1995;46:48–51.
17. Suzuki K, Mizokami M, Lau JYN, et al. Confirmation of hepatitis C virus transmission through needlestick accidents by molecular evolutionary analysis. J Infect Dis 1994;170:1575–8.
18. Höhne M, Schrier E. Roggendorf. Sequence variability in the env-coding region of hepatitis C virus isolated from patients infected during single source outbreak. Arch Virol 1994;137:25–34.

19. Wasley A, Grytdal S, Gallagher K. Surveillance for acute viral hepatitis– United States, 2006. MMWR Surveill Summ 2008;57(SS-2):1–24.
20. Labus B, Sands L, Rowley P, et al. Acute hepatitis C virus infections attributed to unsafe injections at an endoscopy clinic- Nevada, 2007. MMWR Morb Mortal Wkly Rep 2008;57(19):513–7.
21. Thompson ND, Perz JF, Moorman AC, et al. Nonhospital health care-associated hepatitis B and C virus transmission: United States 1998–2008. Ann Intern Med 2009;150:33–9.
22. Puro V, Lanini S. HBV transmission in healthcare settings and safety devices [electronic letter]. Ann Intern Med [Epub Feb 3, 2009].
23. Zeuzem S, Scheuermann EH, Waschk D, et al. Phylogenetic analysis of hepatitis C virus isolates from hemodialysis patients. Kidney Int 1996;49(3):896–902.
24. Chomczynski P, Sacchi N. Single step method of RNA isolation by acid guanidinium thiocyanate-phenol-chloroform extraction. Anal Biochem 1987;162:156–9.
25. Smith DB, Simmons P. Review: molecular epidemiology of hepatitis C virus. J Gastroenterol Hepatol 1997;12:522–7.
26. Schvarcz R, Johansson B, Nyström B, et al. Nosocomial transmission of hepatitis C virus. Infection 1997;25(2):74–7.
27. Bronowicki J-P, Venard V, Botté C, et al. Patient-to-patient transmission of hepatitis C virus during colonoscopy. N Engl J Med 1997;337(4):237–40.
28. Norder H, Bergström A, Uhnoo I, et al. Confirmation of nosocomial transmission of hepatitis C virus by phylogenetic analysis of the NS5-B region. J Clin Microbiol 1998;36(10):3066–9.
29. Widell A, Christensson B, Wiebe T, et al. Epidemiologic and molecular investigation of outbreaks of hepatitis C virus infection on a pediatric oncology service. Ann Intern Med 1999;130(2):130–4.
30. Silini E, Locasciulli A, Santoleri L, et al. Hepatitis C virus infection in a hematology ward: evidence for nosocomial transmission and impact on hematologic disease outcome. Haematologica 2002;87(11):1200–8.
31. Halfon P, Roubicek C, Gerolami V, et al. Use of phylogenetic analysis of hepatitis C virus (HCV) hypervariable region 1 sequences to trace an outbreak of HCV in an autodialysis unit. J Clin Microbiol 2002;40(4):1541–5.
32. González-Candelas F, Bracho MA, Moya A. Molecular epidemiology and forensic genetics: application to a hepatitis C virus transmission event at a hemodialysis unit. J Infect Dis 2003;187(1):352–8.
33. Krause G, Trepka MJ, Whisenhunt RS, et al. Nosocomial transmission of hepatitis C virus associated with the use of multidose saline vials. Infect Control Hosp Epidemiol 2003;24(2):122–7.
34. Tugwell BD, Patel PR, Williams IT, et al. Transmission of hepatitis C virus to several organ and tissue recipients from an antibody-negative donor. Ann Intern Med 2005;143(9):648–54.
35. Macedo de Oliveira A, White KL, Leschinsky DP, et al. An outbreak of hepatitis C virus infections among outpatients at a hematology/oncology clinic. Ann Intern Med 2005;142(11):898–902.
36. Germain J-M, Carbonne A, Thiers V, et al. Patient-to-patient transmission of hepatitis C virus through the use of multidose vials during general anesthesia. Infect Control Hosp Epidemiol 2005;26(9):789–92.
37. Hmaïed F, Ben Mamou M, Dubois M, et al. Determining the source of nosocomial transmission in hemodialysis units in Tunisia by sequencing NS5B and E2 sequences of HCV. J Med Virol 2007;79(8):1089–94.

38. Carneiro MAS, Teles SA, Lampe E, et al. Molecular and epidemiological study of nosocomial transmission of HCV in hemodialysis patients in Brazil. J Med Virol 2007;79(9):1325–33.
39. Spada E, Abbate I, Sicurezza E, et al. Molecular epidemiology of a hepatitis C virus outbreak in a hemodialysis unit in Italy. J Med Virol 2008;80(2):261–7.
40. Pañella H, Rius C, Caylà, et al. Transmission of hepatitis C virus during computed tomography scanning with contrast. Emerg Infect Dis 2008;14(2):333–6.
41. Mizuno Y, Suzuki K, Mori M, et al. Study of needlestick accidents and hepatitis C virus infectiopn in healthcare workers by molecular evolutionary analysis. J Hosp Infect 1997;35:149–54.
42. Esteban JI, Gómez J, Martell M, et al. Transmission of hepatitis C virus by a cardiac surgeon. N Engl J Med 1996;334(9):555–60.
43. Cody SH, Nainan OV, Garfein GS, et al. Hepatitis C virus transmission from an anesthesiologist to a patient. Arch Intern Med 2002;162(11):345–50.
44. Webster GJ, Hallett R, Walley SA, et al. Molecular epidemiology of a large outbreak of hepatitis B linked to autohaemotherapy. Lancet 2000;356:379–84.
45. Bracho MA, Gosalbes MJ, González Moya A, et al. Molecular epidemiology and evolution in an outbreak of fulminant hepatitis B virus. J Clin Microbiol 2006;44:1288–94.
46. Ramalingam S, Leung T, Cairns H, et al. Transmission of hepatitis B virus (genotype E) in a haemodialysis unit. J Clin Virol 2007;40(2):105–9.
47. Harpaz R, Seidlin L, Averhoff FM, et al. Transmission of hepatitis B virus to multiple patients from a surgeon without evidence of inadequate infection control. N Engl J Med 1996;334(9):549–54.
48. Incident Investigation Teams and Others. Transmission of hepatitis B to patients from four infected surgeons without hepatitis e antigen. N Engl J Med 1997;336(3):178–84.
49. Spijkerman IJ, van Doorn LJ, Janssen MH, et al. Transmission of hepatitis B virus from a surgeon to his patients during high-risk and low-risk surgical procedures during 4 years. Infect Control Hosp Epidemiol 2002;23(6):306–12.
50. Magnius LO, Norder H. Subtypes, genotypes and molecular epidemiology of the hepatitis B virus as reflected by sequence variability of the S-gene. Intervirology 1995;38:24–34.
51. Felsenstein J. Confidence limits on phylogenies: an approach using the bootstrap. Evolution 1985;39:783–91.
52. Saitou N, Nei M. The neighbor-joining method: a new method for reconstructing phylogenetic trees. Mol Biol Evol 1987;4:406–25.
53. Fischer GE, Schaefer MK, Labus B, et al. Hepatitis C infections from unsafe injection practices at a Las Vegas, Nevada endoscopy clinic, submitted for publication.
54. Louie RF, Lau MJ, Lee JH, et al. Multicenter study of the prevalence of blood contamination on point-of-care glucose meters and recommendations for controlling contamination. Point of Care 2005;4(4):158–63.
55. Vitale F, Tramuto F, Orlano A, et al. Can the serological status of "anti-HBc alone" be considered a sentinel marker for detection of "occult" HBV infection? J Med Virol 2008;80:577–82.
56. Allos BM, Schaffner W. Transmission of hepatitis B in the health care setting: the elephant in the room or the mouse? [editorial]. J Infect Dis 2007;195(1):1245–7.
57. Quale JM, Landman D, Wallace B, et al. Déjà vu: nosocomial hepatitis B virus transmission and finger-stick monitoring. Am J Med 1998;105(4):296–301.

Health Care– Associated Transmission of Hepatitis B and C Viruses in Hemodialysis Units

Fabrizio Fabrizi, MD[a,b,*], Paul Martin, MD[b]

KEYWORDS

• Hepatitis B virus • Hepatitis C virus • Dialysis
• Antiviral therapy

Liver disease is a significant cause of morbidity and mortality in patients receiving long-term dialysis. This article summarizes the most recent information on epidemiology, clinical significance, and management of infection by hepatitis B (HBV) and hepatitis C (HCV) viruses in this population.

HBV

Controlling the spread of HBV infection within dialysis units has been a major advance in the management of patients with chronic kidney diseases (CKD). The rate of HBV infection in dialysis units in the developed world is currently low but not negligible. A large multicenter survey conducted by the Centers for Disease Control and Prevention (CDC) reported that in 2002, the prevalence of hepatitis B surface antigen (HBsAg) positivity among hemodialysis (HD) patients was 1%, a figure that had not changed substantially during the prior decade.[1] Similarly, the incidence of HBV infection in dialysis patients also had not changed during the prior decade, and in 2002 was 0.12%.[1]

This work was supported by the grant Project Glomerulonephritis in memory of Pippo Neglia.
[a] Division of Nephrology, Maggiore Hospital, IRCCS Foundation, Pad. Croff, Via Commenda 15, Milano 20122, Italy
[b] Division of Hepatology, Department of Medicine, Center for Liver Diseases, Miller School of Medicine, University of Miami, 1500 NW 12th Avenue, Suite 1101-E, 31101, Miami, FL 33136, USA
* Corresponding author. Division of Nephrology, Maggiore Hospital, IRCCS Foundation, Pad. Croff, Via Commenda 15, Milano 20122, Italy.
E-mail address: fabrizi@policlinico.mi.it (F. Fabrizi).

Clin Liver Dis 14 (2010) 49–60
doi:10.1016/j.cld.2009.11.011
1089-3261/10/$ – see front matter © 2010 Elsevier Inc. All rights reserved.

Outbreaks of HBV infection within dialysis units continue, however, to occur.[2-4] The epidemiology of HBV among HD patients in the less developed world is not well known. The main body of information is based on single-center studies with a prevalence of 2% to 20% chronic HBsAg carriers.[5] A recent analysis of registry data on dialysis patients in Asia-Pacific countries (189,663 dialysis patients from seven countries) reported that the prevalence of HBsAg positivity ranged between 1.3% and 14.6%. Incidence data were only available for Thailand and were not statistically significantly different between HD and peritoneal dialysis (PD) patients (0.4% versus 0%).[6]

Higher HBV infection rates within dialysis units in the developing world can be attributed to several factors, such as the higher background prevalence of HBV in the general population and difficulties in following infection control strategies against HBV. These deficiencies are caused, at least in part, by a lack of financial and other resources.

INFECTION CONTROL PROCEDURES AGAINST HBV IN DIALYSIS UNITS

The incidence of acute HBV infection in patients receiving long-term dialysis in the industrialized world has decreased dramatically over the past three decades by the implementation of control practices including standard body fluid precautions and other HD unit procedures. Standard precautions (also known as "universal precautions") include (1) hand washing after contact with blood and other potentially infectious material, (2) use of gloves when in contact with blood or other potentially infectious material, and (3) use of gowns and face shields when exposure to blood and body fluids is anticipated. In addition to these procedures, there are HD unit precautions unique to the HD setting that are more stringent than universal precautions. They indicate that glove use is necessary whenever patients or HD equipment is touched, with no sharing of supplies, instruments, or medications between HD patients including ancillary supply equipment (trays, blood pressure cuffs, clamps, scissors, and other nondisposable items) permitted.[7] Also, the HD-center precautions specify the separation of clean areas (used for handwashing, handling and storage of medications) from contaminated areas (handling blood samples and HD equipment after use), and cleaning and disinfection of nondisposable items, machines, and environmental surfaces between uses. Further, additional precautions to prevent de novo HBV infection in the HD environment are used: monthly serologic testing for HBsAg of all susceptible patients; prompt review of results; physical separation of HBsAg-positive from HBV-susceptible individuals; and cohorting of separate dialysis staff, instruments, supplies, and HD machines used in patients with HBsAg positivity.[7,8] In addition to these infection control procedures, additional factors have contributed to the reduction of HBV infection: screening of blood and blood products for HBV, reduction of blood transfusions needed in dialysis patients because of erythropoietin use, and vaccination against HBV. Since 1982, hepatitis B vaccination has been recommended for all susceptible patients and staff in HD units. Dialysis patients have a suboptimal response to hepatitis B virus vaccine with diminished seroprotection rates compared with healthy subjects. After completion of vaccination, anti-HBs titers (**Table 1**) of responder patients on regular dialysis are low and decline logarithmically over time. The major decline in the transmission of HBV within HD units (between 1976 and 1980), however, antedated the widespread availability of vaccine against HBV.

NATURAL HISTORY OF HBV INFECTION IN DIALYSIS PATIENTS

The natural history of HBV infection in the dialysis population has been poorly characterized because chronic HBV typically progresses slowly and a long follow-up is

Table 1 Tests for HBV		
Tests		Interpretation
HBsAg	Hepatitis B surface antigen	HBV infection
IgM anti-HBc	Antibody to hepatitis B core antigen	Acute or recent HBV infection
IgG anti-HBc	Antibody to hepatitis B core antigen	Chronic or remote HBV infection
HBsAb	Antibody to hepatitis B surface antigen	Immunity to HBV (vaccine induced or a result of prior infection)
HBeAg	Hepatitis B e antigen	Active replication
HBV DNA	HBV viremia	Active replication

needed to assess the major complications of chronic HBV infection, most notably cirrhosis and hepatocellular carcinoma. In contrast, the life expectancy of patients on long-term dialysis is shorter than in the general population. Additional factors make it difficult to assess HBV-related liver disease in chronic uremia, such as serum aminotransferase values are spuriously low and there is only limited information available on histologic findings. The latter in part reflects the reluctance of clinicians to perform liver biopsies in the CKD population for a variety of reasons including impaired platelet aggregation in chronic uremia. A number of oral agents are now licensed for the treatment of chronic HBV infection; recent recommendations[9] support the use of antiviral treatment in HBV-infected dialysis patients, which further limits the ability to understand progression of liver disease in this population.

The most frequent causes of death among dialysis patients remain cardiovascular disease and sepsis. A multicenter survey has shown that the risk of hepatocellular carcinoma is significantly higher in patients on dialysis, compared with the general population; the standardized incidence ratio was 1.5 (95% confidence interval [CI], 1.5–1.7).[10] This has been linked to the greater prevalence of chronic HBV and hepatitis C infection. Cirrhosis is not frequently recognized in the dialysis population (3%) of the industrialized world, but the death rate for dialysis patients with cirrhosis is 35% higher than those without cirrhosis.[11] A retrospective survey on 787 patients with end-stage kidney disease (384 kidney transplant and 403 HD patients) receiving treatment in Serbia[12] demonstrated that HBsAg-positive HD status was an independent predictor of lowered 15-year survival (odds ratio = 1.904; 95% CI, 1.39–2.61).

HBV-RELATED LIVER DISEASE IN DIALYSIS: BIOCHEMICAL EVIDENCE

Patients on maintenance dialysis with chronic HBsAg carriage typically have modest or absent elevation of aminotransferase levels, are anicteric, and rarely develop symptoms of hepatitis. Serum aminotransferase values are usually depressed in CKD patients (both on dialysis and with less advanced kidney failure), although the reasons underlying this phenomenon are unclear. HBV infection does cause hepatocellular injury in patients on long-term dialysis even if it seems often asymptomatic and indolent. A retrospective study of 727 patients on long-term dialysis in northern Italy demonstrated that mean aminotransferase levels were significantly higher in HBsAg-positive HBV DNA–positive than HBsAg-negative patients on dialysis; AST, 22.86 ± 31.34 versus 14.19 ± 9.7 IU/L ($P = .00001$); and ALT, 25.07 ± 41.59 versus 13.9 ± 41.59 IU/L ($P = .0001$). Multivariate analysis showed a significant and independent association between detectable HBsAg–HBV DNA in serum and AST ($P = .0001$) and ALT ($P = .0001$) activity.[13]

In a cross-sectional study of 757 patients receiving regular HD in Italy, elevated γ-glutamyl transpeptidase levels were independently associated with seropositivity for HBsAg or anti-HCV antibody. Raised γ-glutamyl transpeptidase levels were observed in 22% (41 of 184) of dialysis patients with chronic viral hepatitis, probably a reflection of subtle bile duct injury. The measurement of γ-glutamyl transpeptidase levels may be useful in recognizing liver disease in the dialysis population.[14]

THERAPY OF HEPATITIS B IN DIALYSIS PATIENTS

Only five studies to date have evaluated efficacy and safety of a short course (12 months) of initial monotherapy with lamivudine in 38 patients on long-term HD.[5] Serum HBV DNA rapidly fell below the limit of detection by hybridization assay and ALT became normal in almost all patients. Most patients (21 [62%] of 34) lost HBeAg. No information on histologic improvement during therapy or sustained virologic and biochemical response rates was available. No adverse events attributable to lamivudine were reported. Successful treatment by lamivudine in a patient with decompensated HBV-related cirrhosis undergoing regular HD was also reported.[15] More information is needed on the role of newer antiviral agents, such as entecavir and tenofovir, to treat HBV in this population.

HCV: EPIDEMIOLOGY

With first- and second-generation serologic testing for HCV available, a number of investigators in 1990s reported a high prevalence of anti-HCV seropositivity in patients on maintenance dialysis. Effective screening of blood and blood products virtually eliminated HCV transmission by blood transfusions a decade ago, and a subsequent decline in HCV incidence and prevalence within HD units in developed countries occurred. The latest survey by the CDC indicated that the prevalence of anti-HCV among patients on chronic HD in the United States in 2002 was 7.8% (N = 164,845); the anti-HCV rate had been 10.4% in 1995.[1] A multicenter survey showed that the prevalence of anti–HCV-positive patients dropped from 13.5% (1991) to 6.8% (2000) in a Belgian cohort (N = 1710); prevalence also decreased in many countries, such as France (42%–30%) and Italy (20%–16%).[16]

In spite of the elimination of posttransfusion HCV in chronic dialysis patients, de novo HCV is still frequent among patients undergoing maintenance dialysis in developed countries.[17] Izopet and colleagues[18] performed a large prospective study on 1323 patients on regular HD in France and found an incidence of acute HCV of 0.4% per annum. Outbreaks of HCV infection in dialysis centers of developed countries continue to be reported.[17]

The literature on prevalence and incidence rates of HCV among patients on long-term dialysis in developing countries is much less abundant and is mostly based on small-sized surveys. Important information has been provided by the Asia-Pacific Dialysis Registry data (N = 201,590), which reported HCV seroprevalence ranging between 0.7% and 18.1% across 10 different regions and areas.[6] Prevalence and incidence rates were higher in HD compared with PD population; incidence ratio PD versus HD was 0.33 (95% CI, 0.13–0.75). These reports from less-developed countries suggest that even higher prevalence and incidence rates of HCV are common. This is probably related to nosocomial transmission of HCV within dialysis units, incomplete anti-HCV screening of blood and blood products, and a higher prevalence of HCV in the general population.

NOSOCOMIAL TRANSMISSION OF HCV IN DIALYSIS

Transfusions before blood donor screening for anti-HCV undoubtedly caused many cases of HCV in dialysis units. The occurrence of nosocomial transmission of HCV among patients on maintenance HD is supported by several epidemiologic findings: an independent association between time on dialysis and HCV seroprevalence, the relationship between prevalence and incidence of anti-HCV in individual HD units, a higher frequency of anti-HCV seropositivity in patients on HD at a HD center compared with patients on PD and home-HD treatment, and the relative homogeneity of HCV isolates in patients receiving treatment in the same dialysis unit. The small but definite incidence of acute HCV infection detected in chronic HD patients in developed countries, after the elimination of posttransfusional HCV, also lends support to the possibility of HCV transmission by nosocomial route.[19]

The occurrence of nosocomial transmission was confirmed when phylogenetic analysis identified clusters of closely related isolates of HCV, both in studies of individual units with high seroconversion rates and multicenter surveys.[19] Parts of the HCV genome, especially hypervariable region 1, are highly variable and lend themselves to fingerprinting of each isolate or quasispecies using nucleic acid sequencing. This may be used to establish a firm basis for studies of spread and routes of HCV infection.

MODES OF NOSOCOMIAL TRANSMISSION OF HCV IN DIALYSIS UNITS

Since the dramatic reduction in the 1990s of the risk of posttransfusional HCV, nosocomial transmission is currently the usual source when HD patients seroconvert to anti-HCV positivity. The most likely cause of HCV transmission between patients treated in the same dialysis unit is cross-contamination from supplies and surface (including gloves) as a result of failure to follow infection-control procedures within the unit. Other possible transmission routes are direct contact between patients, a common infected blood donor, or invasive procedures outside using contaminated instruments.

A systematic review of molecular virology papers that included both confirmation of the source patients and an investigation of possible transmission routes suggested that the internal HD machine circuit is, at most, a minor contributor to the nosocomial transmission of HCV among HD patients.[20] There is no reason to believe that a publication bias has suppressed the reporting of nosocomial transmission related to the dialysis equipment or favored reporting of transmission because of breaches in infection control procedures.

Dialyzer reuse was not identified as a risk factor for seroconversion for HCV in the CDC surveillance data.[1] In the United States multicenter database (DOOPS), seroconversion was not significantly associated with dialyzer reuse (relative risk 0.70; $P = .15$).[21]

The CDC does not currently recommend designated machines or patient isolation to prevent nosocomial transmission of HCV within HD units; a ban on dialyzer reuse has not been advocated.[7] Similar recommendations were expressed in the recently published Kidney Disease Improving Global Outcomes statements.[22] No randomized controlled trials exist on the impact of isolation on the risk of transmission of HCV to HD patients; however, two large prospective observational studies have demonstrated that isolation does not protect against HCV transmission in HD patients.[21,23] By logistic regression analysis, the increased risk for HCV infection was not diminished by isolation of HCV-infected patients (relative risk = 1.01; $P = .99$) in the DOPPS survey.[21]

Although prospective trials have shown a reduction in HCV transmission within dialysis units by complete isolation of anti–HCV-seropositive patients, none have included a control group.[24–28] It remains unclear whether the reported improvement resulted from adoption of an isolation policy or rather from the simultaneous reinforcement of the application of infection control procedures. Some prospective observational studies have reported a reduction of HCV transmission after the reinforcement of basic hygienic precautions, without any isolation measures.[29] In particular, some investigators have been able to reduce the yearly incidence of anti-HCV seroconversion to 0% by enforcement of infection control measures against blood-borne pathogens.[30,31] This suggests that prevention of HCV transmission within HD units is possible in the absence of any isolation policy.

Current infection control procedures to prevent HCV transmission in dialysis units include universal precautions and routine HD unit precautions. Periodic anti-HCV antibody testing for infection control purposes within dialysis units is currently recommended by CDC.

NATURAL HISTORY OF HCV INFECTION IN DIALYSIS UNITS

There is some information on the association between anti-HCV seropositive serologic status and survival in patients on maintenance HD. The quality of evidence is generally low. An accurate assessment of the natural history of HCV in the dialysis population has been difficult to obtain. The natural history of HCV infection extends over decades rather than years, whereas dialysis patients have higher morbidity and mortality rates than those of the general population because of age and comorbid conditions, making the long-term consequences of HCV infection difficult to establish. Aminotransferase values are typically lower in the dialysis than in nonuremic populations. Dialysis patients who have detectable serum HCV RNA have aminotransferase levels greater than those who do not, although values are typically within the "normal" range.[19] In addition, recent advances in antiviral therapy for hepatitis C support antiviral treatment of HCV in the CKD population in at least some instances; this hampers the implementation of large trials on the natural history of HCV in this population.

A recent meta-analysis of observational studies involving 11,589 unique patients on maintenance dialysis demonstrated that the presence of anti-HCV antibody was an independent and significant risk factor for death; the summary estimate for adjusted relative risk (all-cause mortality) was 1.34 (95% CI, 1.13–1.59).[32] Liver dysfunction has been implicated in a lower survival of seropositive patients; the summary estimate for relative risk of liver-related mortality was 5.89 (95% CI, 1.93–17.99). These data are in keeping with other sources[33,34]; the presence of anti-HCV antibody was an independent predictor of mortality (relative risk, 1.37; 95% CI, 1.15–1.62; $P = .003$) in the Japanese HD cohort, according to the Asia-Pacific Dialysis Registry data.[6]

THERAPY OF HEPATITIS C IN DIALYSIS POPULATION

The benefits and risks of antiviral therapy with interferon (IFN)-based regimen in HCV-infected patients on maintenance HD have been evaluated in several studies of appropriate size.[35,36] A meta-analysis identified 24 clinical trials enrolling 429 unique patients on maintenance dialysis who received conventional IFN monotherapy; the summary estimate for sustained virologic response rate was 39% (95% CI, 32–46) and drop-out rate was 19% (95% CI, 13–26).[36] The studies were heterogeneous with regard to sustained virologic response and drop-out rate. No publication bias was found. The conclusion of the authors was that one third of dialysis patients with chronic hepatitis C were successfully treated with conventional IFN monotherapy.

The viral response to monotherapy with standard IFN in maintenance HD patients (summary estimate of 39%) is higher than that observed in patients with chronic hepatitis C and normal kidney function (7%–16%) who received conventional IFN monotherapy.[37,38] Several mechanisms account for the relatively higher response to IFN in patients receiving regular HD. Dialysis patients with HCV usually have a lower viral load, the infection is frequently associated with milder forms of liver disease, clearance of IFN is lower in dialysis than in non-CKD patients, and an increase in endogenous IFN release from circulating white blood cells during HD procedures has been reported.[39] A marked and prolonged synthesis of hepatocyte growth factor (or other cytokines) caused by HD may play an additional role.[40]

Although response rates to conventional IFN are better in the dialysis population, tolerance to IFN monotherapy seems lower in patients on maintenance HD than in non-CKD individuals. The summary estimate for drop-out rate was 19% in dialysis patients who received standard IFN monotherapy, whereas the frequency of side effects requiring IFN discontinuation ranged between 5% and 9% in non-CKD patients with chronic hepatitis C who received IFN monotherapy (3 MUI thrice weekly for 6 months).[37,38] The most frequent side effects requiring interruption of treatment in dialysis patients after antiviral therapy were flulike symptoms and gastrointestinal and hematologic abnormalities. A relationship between age and drop-out rate was found, even if no statistical significance was reached ($P = .064$).[36] The altered pharmacokinetic parameters of IFN in the HD population may, to some extent, explain the higher frequency of side effects leading to IFN discontinuation. IFN-alpha half-life was longer in dialysis than in normal controls (9.6 versus 5.3 hours; $P = .001$) with an area under the curve twice that of patients with normal kidney function.[41] Additional mechanisms were older age and high rate of comorbid conditions in HD population.[5]

COMBINATION THERAPY FOR HEPATITIS C IN DIALYSIS

The current standard of care for HCV infection in patients with normal renal function is combined antiviral therapy (pegylated IFN plus ribavirin). The long-acting pegylated IFNs, because of their longer half-life, are administrated as a weekly dose. A single-dose study in patients with stable chronic renal failure found no significant difference between patients with normal and diminished kidney function.[42] In a separate analysis, it was reported that HD had negligible effects on pegylated IFN alpha-2b clearance.[43] The pharmacokinetics of pegylated IFN during HD may vary in the dialysis population, depending on the permeability and dialyzer pore use.[44]

Data on monotherapy with pegylated IFN in dialysis patients with HCV are mostly based on small and uncontrolled clinical trials[45–59]; it seems that pegylated IFN does not increase viral response in comparison with conventional IFN. Information on combined antiviral therapy (ie, conventional IFN plus ribavirin) in CKD population is very preliminary in nature[60,61] and the data on pegylated IFN with ribavirin are even more sparse.[62–67] The quality of evidence on this issue is generally very low. The results given in some trials have been encouraging in terms of efficacy (**Table 2**) and safety, but the limited size of the study groups does not allow definitive conclusions.

Very little ribavirin is removed by dialysis so there is a propensity for drug to accumulate, with hemolysis in the dialysis population already at significant risk for anemia. Ribavirin therapy in this setting is not recommended. If a decision is made to use ribavirin in patients on maintenance HD, it should be used very cautiously and only after the implementation of several precautions, including (1) very low doses of ribavirin (200 mg daily or thrice weekly); (2) weekly monitoring of hemoglobin levels; and

Table 2
Pegylated interferon in combination with ribavirin in patients with chronic hepatitis C on maintenance hemodialysis: clinical trials

Authors	% SVR	Antiviral Agent
Bruchfeld A, et al, 2006	50 (3/6)	Peg-IFN alfa-2a (N = 2) or peg-IFN alfa-2b (N = 4) plus ribavirin
Rendina M, et al, 2007	97 (34/35)	Peg-IFN alfa-2a plus ribavirin
[a]Schmitz V, et al, 2007	50 (3/6)	Peg-IFN alfa-2b plus ribavirin
Carriero D, et al, 2008	29 (4/14)	Peg-IFN alfa-2a plus ribavirin
Van Leusen R, et al, 2008	71 (4/7)	Peg-IFN alfa-2a plus ribavirin
[b]Liu CH, et al, 2009	60 (21/35)	Peg-IFN alfa-2a plus ribavirin

Results have been calculated according to an intention to-treat analysis.
Abbreviations: IFN, interferon; SVR, sustained virologic response.
[a] This study concerned liver-kidney transplant recipients.
[b] Only relapser patients after IFN monotherapy were included.

(3) high doses of erythropoietin to treat anemia.[22] Adequate iron stores to boost erythropoietin activity are required. A tentative safe therapeutic range of ribavirin trough plasma concentration of 10 to 15 μmol/L has been proposed.[62] This typically is performed at specialized centers.

Overall, there is concern about the applicability of these studies to all dialysis patients because most of the subjects included in these studies were on the waiting list for kidney transplantation and were younger and probably healthier than the general dialysis population. Furthermore, only a minority of studies were from North America where many CKD patients are African American. This is of special relevance, because there are racial differences in the response to IFN therapy in subjects with normal kidney function.[68]

SUMMARY

Prevention of nosocomial transmission of HBV has been a signal achievement in the management of CKD. The rate of serum HBsAg seropositivity in patients on maintenance HD in the developed world is currently low but outbreaks of acute HBV continue to occur. The prevalence of HBV infection within dialysis units in developing countries is higher. Although data are limited, HBV infection in dialysis population diminishes survival. No controlled clinical trials for treatment of hepatitis B with IFN or lamivudine therapy in dialysis patients are currently available. HCV remains common in patients undergoing regular dialysis and is an important cause of liver disease in this population. Anti-HCV screening of blood products has almost eliminated posttransfusion HCV infection but acquisition of HCV continues to occur in dialysis patients because of nosocomial spread. Recent data show that HCV has a detrimental role on survival of chronic dialysis patients. The response rate to conventional IFN monotherapy may be higher in dialysis patients than those with normal kidney function but tolerance is lower. Only limited data about pegylated IFN alone or in association with ribavirin for hepatitis C in dialysis population exist.

REFERENCES

1. Finelli L, Miller JT, Tokars JI, et al. National surveillance of dialysis-associated diseases in the United States, 2002. Semin Dial 2005;18:52–61.

2. Kondili LA, Genovese D, Argentini C, et al. Nosocomial transmission in simultaneous outbreaks of hepatitis C and B virus infections in a hemodialysis center. Eur J Clin Microbiol Infect Dis 2006;25:527–31.
3. Inoue K, Ogawa O, Yamada M, et al. Possible association of vigorous hepatitis B virus replication with the development of fulminant hepatitis. J Gastroenterol 2006;41:383–7.
4. Burdick RA, Bragg-Gresham JL, Woods JD, et al. Patterns of hepatitis B prevalence and seroconversion in hemodialysis units from three continents: the DOPPS. Kidney Int 2003;63:2222–9.
5. Fabrizi F, Messa PG, Martin P. Hepatitis B virus infection and the dialysis patient. Semin Dial 2008;21:440–6.
6. Johnson DW, Dent H, Yao Q, et al. Frequencies of hepatitis B and C infections among haemodialysis and peritoneal dialysis patients in Asia-Pacific countries: analysis of registry data. Nephrol Dial Transplant. doi: 10.1093/ndt/gfn 684, 2008. [Epub ahead of print].
7. Center for Disease Control and Prevention. Recommendations for preventing transmission of infections among chronic hemodialysis patients. MMWR Recomm Rep 2001;50:1–43.
8. Kellerman S, Alter MJ. Preventing hepatitis B and hepatitis C virus infection in end-stage renal disease patients: back to basics. Hepatology 1999;29:291–3.
9. Marzano A, Angelucci E, Andreone P, et al. Italian Association for the Study of the Liver (AISF). Prophylaxis and treatment of hepatitis B in immunocompromised patients. Dig Liver Dis 2007;39:397–408.
10. Maisonneuve P, Agodoa L, Gellert R, et al. Cancer in patients on dialysis for end-stage renal disease: an international collaborative study. Lancet 1999;354:93–9.
11. Marcelli D, Stanhard D, Conte F, et al. ESRD patient mortality with adjustment for comorbid conditions in Lombardy (Italy) versus the United States. Kidney Int 1996;50:1013–8.
12. Visnja L, Milan S, Jelena M, et al. Hepatitis B and hepatitis C virus infection and outcome of hemodialysis and kidney transplant patients. Ren Fail 2008;30:81–7.
13. Fabrizi F, Mangano S, Alongi G, et al. Influence of hepatitis B virus viremia upon serum aminotransferase activity in dialysis population. Int J Artif Organs 2003;26:1048–55.
14. Fabrizi F, De Vecchi AF, Qureshi AR, et al. Gammaglutamyltranspeptidase activity and viral hepatitis in dialysis patients. Int J Artif Organs 2007;30:6–15.
15. Komorizono Y, Uchida Y, Sako K, et al. Successful treatment by lamivudine and regular hemodialysis in a patient with decompensated hepatitis B virus-related cirrhosis complicated by terminal renal impairment. J Clin Gastroenterol 2004;38:831–2.
16. Jadoul M, Poignet JL, Geddes C, et al. The changing epidemiology of hepatitis C virus (HCV) infection in hemodialysis: European multicentre study. Nephrol Dial Transplant 2004;19:904–9.
17. Thompson ND, Perz JF, Moorman AC, et al. Nonhospital health-care associated hepatitis B and C virus transmission: United States, 1998–2008. Ann Intern Med 2009;150:33–9.
18. Izopet J, Sandres-Saune' K, Kamar N, et al. Incidence of HCV infection in French hemodialysis units: a prospective study. J Med Virol 2005;77:70–6.
19. Fabrizi F, Lunghi G, Ganeshan V, et al. Hepatitis C virus infection and the dialysis patient. Semin Dial 2007;20:416–22.
20. Fabrizi F, Messa P, Martin P. Transmission of hepatitis C virus infection in haemodialysis: current concepts. Int J Artif Organs 2008;31:1004–16.

21. Fissell RB, Bragg-Gresham JL, Woods JD, et al. Patterns of hepatitis C prevalence and seroconversion in hemodialysis units from three continents: the DOPPS. Kidney Int 2004;65:2335–42.
22. Kidney Disease. Improving global outcomes: KDIGO clinical practice guidelines for the prevention, diagnosis, evaluation, and treatment of hepatitis C in chronic kidney disease. Kidney Int 2008;73(Suppl 109):S1–99.
23. Petrosillo N, Gilli P, Serraino D, et al. Prevalence of infected patients and understaffing have a role in hepatitis C virus transmission in dialysis. Am J Kidney Dis 2001;37:1004–10.
24. Blumberg A, Zehnder C, Burckhardt JJ. Prevention of hepatitis C infection in haemodialysis units: a prospective study. Nephrol Dial Transplant 1995;10: 230–3.
25. Djordjevic V, Stojanovic K, Stojanovic M, et al. Prevention of nosocomial transmission of hepatitis C infection in a hemodialysis unit: a prospective study. Int J Artif Organs 2000;23:181–8.
26. Taskapan H, Oymak O, Dogukan A, et al. Patient to patient transmission of hepatitis C virus in hemodialysis units. Clin Nephrol 2001;55:477–81.
27. Arenas DJ, Paya S, Gonzalez C, et al. Isolation of HCV patients is efficient in reducing the annual incidence of HCV infection, but is it really necessary? [letter]. Nephrol Dial Transplant 1999;14:1337–9.
28. Gallego E, Lopez A, Perez J, et al. Effect of isolation measures on the incidence and prevalence of hepatitis C virus infection in hemodialysis. Nephron Clin Pract 2006;104:c1–6.
29. Valtuille R, Moretto H, Lef L, et al. Decline of high hepatitis C virus prevalence in a hemodialysis unit with no isolation measures during a 6-year follow-up. Clin Nephrol 2002;57:371–5.
30. Gilli P, Soffritti S, De Paoli Vitali E, et al. Prevention of hepatitis C virus in dialysis units. Nephron 1995;70:301–6.
31. Jadoul M, Cornu C, van Ypersele de Strihou C, The Universitaries Cliniques St-Luc (UCL) Collaborative Group. Universal precautions prevent hepatitis C virus transmission: a 54 month follow-up of the Belgian Multicenter Study. Kidney Int 1998;53:10221–5.
32. Fabrizi F, Takkouche B, Lunghi G, et al. The impact of hepatitis C virus infection on survival in dialysis patients: meta-analysis of observational studies. J Viral Hepat 2007;14:697–703.
33. Santoro D, Mazzaglia G, Savica V, et al. Hepatitis status and mortality in hemodialysis population. Ren Fail 2009;31:6–12.
34. Wang SM, Liu JH, Chou CY, et al. Mortality in hepatitis C-positive patients treated with peritoneal dialysis. Perit Dial Int 2008;28:183–7.
35. Russo MW, Goldsweig C, Iacobson M, et al. Interferon monotherapy for dialysis patients with chronic hepatitis C: an analysis of the literature on efficacy and safety. Am J Gastroenterol 2003;98:1610–5.
36. Fabrizi F, Dixit V, Messa P, et al. Interferon monotherapy of chronic hepatitis C in dialysis patients: meta-analysis of clinical trials. J Viral Hepat 2008;15: 79–88.
37. Davis GL, Balart LA, Schiff ER, et al. Treatment of chronic hepatitis C with recombinant interferon alfa: a multicenter randomized, controlled trial. Hepatitis Interventional Therapy Group. N Engl J Med 1989;321:1501–6.
38. Thevenot T, Regimbeau C, Ratziu V, et al. Meta-analysis of interferon randomized trials in the treatment of viral hepatitis C in naïve patients: 1999 update. J Viral Hepat 2001;8:48–62.

39. Badalamenti S, Catania A, Lunghi G, et al. Changes in viremia and circulating interferon-alpha during hemodialysis in hepatitis C virus-positive patients: only coincidental phenomena? Am J Kidney Dis 2003;42:143–50.
40. Rampino T, Arbustini E, Gregorini M, et al. Hemodialysis prevents liver disease caused by hepatitis C virus: role of hepatocyte growth factor. Kidney Int 1999; 56:2286–91.
41. Rostaing L, Chatelut E, Payen JL, et al. Pharmacokinetics of alphaIFN-2b in chronic hepatitis C virus patients undergoing chronic hemodialysis or with normal renal function: clinical implications. J Am Soc Nephrol 1998;9:2344–8.
42. Martin P, Mitra S, Farrington K, et al. Pegylated (40 KD) interferon alfa-2a (Pegasys) is unaffected by renal impairment [abstract]. Hepatology 2000; 32:370A.
43. Gupta SK, Pittenger AL, Swan SK, et al. Single-dose pharmacokinetics and safety of pegylated interferon-alpha2b in patients with chronic renal dysfunction. J Clin Pharmacol 2002;42:1109–15.
44. Barril G, Quiroga JA, Sanz P, et al. Pegylated interferon-alpha2a kinetics during experimental haemodialysis: impact of permeability and pore size of dialyzers. Aliment Pharmacol Ther 2004;20:37–44.
45. Mukherjee S, Gilroy RK, McCashland TM, et al. Pegylated interferon for recurrent hepatitis C in liver transplant recipients with renal failure: a prospective cohort study. Transplant Proc 2003;35:1478–9.
46. Annichiarico BE, Siciliano M. Pegylated interferon alpha-2b monotherapy for hemodialysis patients with chronic hepatitis C [letter]. Aliment Pharmacol Ther 2004;20:123–7.
47. Teta D, Luscher BL, Gonvers JJ, et al. Pegylated interferon for the treatment of hepatitis C virus in haemodialysis patients. Nephrol Dial Transplant 2005;20: 901–3.
48. Covic A, Maftei ID, Mardare NGI, et al. Analysis of safety and efficacy of pegylated-interferon alpha-2a in hepatitis C virus positive hemodialysis patients: results from a large, multicenter audit. J Nephrol 2006;19:794–801.
49. Sporea I, Popescu A, Sirli R, et al. Pegylated interferon alpha2a treatment for chronic hepatitis C in patients on chronic hemodialysis. World J Gastroenterol 2006;16:4191–4.
50. Russo MW, Ghalib R, Sigal S, et al. Randomized trial of pegylated interferon alpha-2b monotherapy in hemodialysis patients with chronic hepatitis C. Nephrol Dial Transplant 2006;21:437–43.
51. Kokoglu OF, Ucmak H, Hosoglu S, et al. Efficacy and tolerability of pegylated-interferon alpha-2a in hemodialysis patients with chronic hepatitis C. J Gastroenterol Hepatol 2006;21:575–80.
52. Casanovas-Taltavull T, Baliellas C, Llobet M, et al. Preliminary results of treatment with pegylated interferon alpha2a for chronic hepatitis C virus in kidney transplant candidates on hemodialysis. Transplant Proc 2007;39:2125–7.
53. Chan TM, Ho SKN, Tang CSO, et al. Pilot study of pegylated interferon-alpha 2a in dialysis patients with chronic hepatitis C virus infection. Nephrology 2007;12: 11–7.
54. Amarapurkar DN, Patel ND, Kirpalani AL. Monotherapy with peginterferon alpha-2b (12kDA) for chronic hepatitis C infection in patients undergoing haemodialysis. Trop Gastroenterol 2007;28:16–8.
55. Liu CH, Liang CC, Lin JW, et al. Pegylated interferon alfa-2a versus standard interferon alfa-2a for treatment-naïve dialysis patients with chronic hepatitis C: a randomised study. Gut 2008;57:525–30.

56. Ayaz C, Celen MK, Yuce UN, et al. Efficacy and safety of pegylated-interferon alpha-2a in hemodialysis patients with chronic hepatitis C. World J Gastroenterol 2008;14:255–9.

57. Akhan SC, Kalender B, Ruzgar M. The response to pegylated interferon alpha 2a in haemodialysis patients with hepatitis C virus infection. Infection 2008;36:341–4.

58. UcMaky H, Kokoglu OF, Hosoglu S, et al. Long-term efficacy of pegylated interferon alpha-2a in HCV-positive hemodialysis patients. Ren Fail 2008;30:227–32.

59. Sikole A, Dzekova P, Selja N, et al. Treatment of hepatitis C in haemodialysis patients with pegylated interferon alpha2a as monotherapy. Ren Fail 2008;29:227–32.

60. Mousa DH, Abdalla AH, Al-Shoail G, et al. Alpha-interferon with ribavirin in the treatment of hemodialysis patients with hepatitis C. Transplant Proc 2004;36:1831–4.

61. Bruchfeld A, Stahle L, Andersson J, et al. Ribavirin treatment in dialysis patients with chronic hepatitis C virus infection: a pilot study. J Viral Hepat 2001;8:287–92.

62. Bruchfeld A, Lindahl K, Reichard O, et al. Pegylated interferon and ribavirin treatment for hepatitis C in hemodialysed patients. J Viral Hepat 2006;13:316–21.

63. Rendina M, Castellaneta NM, Castellaneta A, et al. The treatment of chronic hepatitis C with peginterferon alpha2a (40 kDA) plus ribavirin in hemodialysed patients awaiting renal transplant. J Hepatol 2007;46:764–8.

64. Schmitz V, Kiessling A, Bahra M, et al. Peginterferon alfa-2b plus ribavirin for the treatment of hepatitis C recurrence following combined liver and kidney transplantation. Ann Transplant 2007;12:22–7.

65. van Leusen R, Adang RP, de Vries RA, et al. Pegylated interferon alfa-2a (40KD) and ribavirin in haemodialysis patients with chronic hepatitis C. Nephrol Dial Transplant 2008;23:721–5.

66. Carriero D, Fabrizi F, Uriel A, et al. Treatment of dialysis patients with chronic hepatitis C using pegylated-interferon and low dose ribavirin. Int J Artif Organs 2008;31:295–302.

67. Liu CH, Liang CC, Tsai HB, et al. Pegylated interferon alpha-2a plus low-dose ribavirin for the retreatment of dialysis chronic hepatitis C patients who relapsed from prior interferon monotherapy. Gut 2009;58:314–6.

68. Rodriguez-Torres M, Jeffers LJ, Sheikh MY, et al. Peginterferon alfa-2a and ribavirin in Latino and non-Latino whites with hepatitis C. N Engl J Med 2009;360:257–67.

Health Care–Associated Transmission of Hepatitis B and C Viruses in Endoscopy Units

Hao Wu, MB[a], Bo Shen, MD[b],*

KEYWORDS

- Hepatitis B • Hepatitis C • Gastrointestinal endoscopy
- Endoscopy-related infection

The risk for potential transmission of infectious agents during gastrointestinal (GI) endoscopy is concerning for patients and physicians. For example, a recent news report on possible infection transmission during colonoscopies and other procedures in a few Veterans Affairs (VA) facilities in the Southeastern United States drew tremendous media attention and public panic. The VA recently warned some veterans who had colonoscopies as far back as 5 years ago that they may have been exposed to the body fluids of other patients and should undergo tests to make sure they have not contracted serious illnesses.[1] However, the instance of infection transmission remains rare after GI endoscopy procedures, with an estimated frequency of 1 in 1.8 million procedures.[2] Endoscopy-related infection may occur when microorganisms are spread or transmitted from patient to patient by contaminated endoscopic or accessory equipments; from the GI tract through the bloodstream during endoscopy to susceptible organs or prostheses, or spread to adjacent tissues that are breached as a result of the endoscopy procedure; or from patients to endoscopy personnel and perhaps from endoscopy personnel to patients.[3]

Nosocomial transmission of microorganisms, including hepatitis viruses, during GI an endoscopy procedure is often associated with inadequately reprocessed endoscopes, insufficiently disinfection of endoscopes, failure to autoclave reusable

a Department of Gastroenterology, Zhongshan Hospital, Fudan University, Shanghai, China
b Digestive Disease Institute-A31, Cleveland Clinic, 9500 Euclid Avenue, Cleveland, OH 44195, USA
* Corresponding author.
E-mail address: shenb@ccf.org (B. Shen).

Clin Liver Dis 14 (2010) 61–68
doi:10.1016/j.cld.2009.11.012
1089-3261/10/$ – see front matter © 2010 Elsevier Inc. All rights reserved.

liver.theclinics.com

accessories after each use, or improper sharing of multidose vials of intravenous medications.[4,5] Spach and colleagues[2] reviewed the literature between 1966 and 1992 and documented 281 reported cases of transmission of microorganisms by GI endoscopy, including hepatitis viruses. The vast majority of these cases occurred before the adoption of the initial 1988 guidelines that emphasized the need for thorough manual cleaning of endoscopes before disinfection.[6] Only 28 cases of transmission of infection that were associated with endoscopy procedures were reported between 1988 and 1992, with an estimated 40 million GI endoscopies performed over the same period. However, the actual prevalence of infection transmission might have been higher, as there might have been underreporting, unrecognized asymptomatic infections, or unrecognized association of infections with prior endoscopy. Nonetheless, with the adoption of the stringent 2003 multi-society guidelines,[7] the transmission rate of infection by GI endoscopy may be even lower.[8]

Although GI endoscopic procedures have been implicated in the transmission of viral infections, including hepatitis C (HCV) and hepatitis B (HBV),[9] the establishment of a causal relationship between GI endoscopy procedures and viral transmission can be difficult, as acute viral infections, such as with HCV and HBV, are usually asymptomatic and have a long period of incubation. Therefore, linking transmission of these infections to a procedure done in the past may be difficult.

TRANSMISSION OF HEPATITIS C DURING GASTROINTESTINAL ENDOSCOPY

HCV transmission in the health care setting is a major mode of global spread, with the World Health Organization Global Burden of Disease study estimating that in 2000, contaminated injections led to 2 million HCV infections, or 40% of new infections worldwide.[10] Endoscopy procedures as a vehicle for HCV transmission have been suspected since 1996, when blood banks in France and Italy suspended donors who reported a history of recent digestive endoscopy from donating blood for 6 months and up to 1 year, respectively.[11] Up to 2003, a comprehensive review of the published literature and the US Food and Drug Administration database found only 35 confirmed cases of transmission of infection during GI endoscopy in the prior decade.[12] An estimated HCV infection rate approaches 1 per 10 million procedures. Whether a GI endoscopy procedure poses an increased risk for transmission of HCV is still controversial. It is generally thought that in many instances the link between endoscopy procedure and infection may be caused by an improperly processed endoscope, inadequate aseptic techniques, and an improper administration of intravenous medications.

Early case reports and epidemiologic studies suggested an association between GI endoscopy and HCV seropositivity. There are case reports of transmission of HCV during GI endoscopies in the 1990s,[13,14] in a setting where lapses in high level disinfection of endoscopes have occurred. Bronowicki and colleagues[14] documented transmission of HCV from an infected patient to two subsequent patients who underwent colonoscopy procedures using the same endoscope. Transmission was attributed to breaches in endoscope reprocessing (ie, failure to mechanically clean the working channel of the endoscope before disinfection, and failure to sterilize the biopsy forceps between patients). In addition, inadequate aseptic techniques practiced at this center also raised the possibility of transmission of the virus by way of contaminated intravenous tubing, syringes, or multidose vials rather than the colonoscope instrument itself. In early 2008, the US Center for Disease Control (CDC) received a report from the Southern Nevada Health District concerning surveillance reports regarding two individuals newly diagnosed with acute hepatitis C. A third person with acute hepatitis C was reported the following day. This report raised concerns about an outbreak because the health district typically confirms four or fewer cases of acute hepatitis C per year. Initial inquiries found that all three persons with acute hepatitis C underwent procedures at the same endoscopy clinic within 35 to 90 days of illness onset. A joint investigation with CDC was initiated. The epidemiologic and laboratory investigation revealed that HCV transmission likely resulted from reuse of syringes on individual patients and use of single-use medication vials on multiple patients at the clinic.[5]

A case-control study of incident HCV infection was conducted to identify persistent modes of transmission in France, involving repeat blood donors who seroconverted between 1998 and 2001 and seroconverters referred to hepatology departments in 2000 through 2001. For each subject, four age- and sex-matched controls were randomly selected from the population of occurrence. Sixty-four subjects and 227 controls were included. A multivariate analysis showed that having had a GI endoscopy was an independent risk factor with an adjusted odds ratio of 5.7 (95% CI, 1.4–23.8).[15] Community-based, cross-sectional studies of risk factors for HCV infection in rural Egyptian villages showed that subjects who had had an upper endoscopy were more likely to have had anti-HCV than age-matched controls not having the procedure.[16,17] Among 22 of 3999 inhabitants who had an upper endoscopy in a Nile Delta village, the odds ratio for having anti-HCV with was 1.4 (not statistically significant) as compared with an overall anti-HCV prevalence of 24%.[16] In a larger population, 6012 inhabitants of a village with 9% HCV prevalence, the age-adjusted association of endoscopy with anti-HCV positivity was statistically significant (odds ratio of 6.2 among those 30 years old or younger and odds ratio of 1.7 in those more than 30 years old).[17]

Caution should be taken when results of these epidemiology or cross-sectional studies are interpreted. Reporting biases may have existed when there was a reliance on self reporting of risk factors for HCV (with confounding factors, such as intravenous drug abuse and history of blood transfusion).[18] In most instances, it is not clear whether endoscope reprocessing protocols were followed during the study period; whether general infection control practices (eg, reuse of syringes or multiple-dose vials) were adhered to; or even whether endoscopy preceded the diagnosis of HCV infection.[19] Furthermore, patients infected with HCV could have had their upper endoscopy from a complication of HCV, such as liver cirrhosis.

Subsequent studies on the effectiveness of the usual disinfection procedures in eliminating HCV particles indicate that all anecdotal cases of endoscopic HCV transmission could be attributed to breaches in recommended regimens.[20–22] The viral transmission is extremely rare in GI endoscopy if guidelines are strictly obeyed. Proper cleaning, processing, and disinfection of endoscopy instruments appear to have a positive impact on the prevention of HCV infection transmission. Studies have indicated that when currently accepted reprocessing guidelines are followed, endoscopy-related transmission of HCV did not occur. In a prospective study from three endoscopy centers and two blood banks in Northern Italy, 9008 subjects were tested negative for anti-HCV antibody and 8260 (92%) were retested for anti-HCV 6 months after endoscopy. All units participating in this study adhered to the guidelines for cleaning and disinfection practices in digestive endoscopy and reprocessing endoscopic accessories. The control group consisted of 51,230 unexposed, healthy, anti-HCV–negative persons who donated blood at two blood banks in the same area and during the same time period; 38,280 of them (75%) were tested again for anti-HCV 6 to 48 months after the first blood donation. All 8260 subjects undergoing endoscopy remained negative for anti-HCV 6 months after the procedure. None of the

912 subjects who underwent endoscopy with the same instrument previously used on HCV carriers showed anti-HCV seroconversion. In contrast, four blood donors in the control group became positive for anti-HCV or HCV RNA.[23] The instruments used for the known HCV carriers were not handled differently from those used for the HCV-negative subjects; they were not removed from the general instrument pool, were disinfected in the same way as the others, and were then used promptly to perform endoscopy on the HCV-negative subjects.[23] These findings suggest that properly performed endoscopy is not a major risk factor for HCV transmission. This notion is further supported by a prospective cohort study from Egypt. The incidence of HCV and HBV cross infections was conducted in an endoscopic unit at a specialty liver hospital in Egypt. A total of 859 subjects, including 149 of 249 subjects (60%) at risk (anti-HCV negative), were retested 3 to 10 months after the upper endoscopy with endoscopes previously used on HCV carriers. The endoscopes were properly cleaned, disinfected, and processed following the American Society for Gastrointestinal Endoscopy (ASGE) and the Society of Gastroenterology Nurses and Associates guidelines. Four subjects, initially negative, tested positive for anti-HCV antibody with enzyme immunoassays after the upper endoscopy. However, two of these subjects had HCV-RNA in their baseline blood samples, and the other two did not have HCV-RNA in their follow-up samples. There were no cases of proven transmission of HCV when endoscopes were reprocessed by using currently accepted standards.[24] This study confirms the notion that transmission of HCV through the digestive endoscopy is minimal, as long as the guidelines are strictly followed. Together these studies indicate that when currently accepted guidelines for cleaning and disinfection of endoscopes are followed, transmission of HCV through endoscopes does not, or only rarely, occur.

TRANSMISSION OF HEPATITIS B DURING GASTROINTESTINAL ENDOSCOPY

Transmission of HBV during GI endoscopy is not well documented.[6] A few isolated case reports have suggested that transmission of HBV is possible when endoscopes are inadequately reprocessed.[25–27] Five prospective studies followed 120 subjects who had undergone endoscopy with an instrument previously used in HBV-infected subjects.[28–32] No subjects who were HBV-seronegative developed clinical or serologic evidence of hepatitis B over a 6-month follow-up. In another set of prospective studies, a total of 722 subjects who were HBV-seronegative were followed for up to 12 months after endoscopy, with background prevalence rates of hepatitis B surface antigen (HBsAg) positivity in these populations of up to 9.6%.[33–36] Despite minimal disinfection of the endoscopes between procedures, only three subjects were seroconverted. None of the seroconversions were thought to be related to the endoscopy procedure because none of these subjects had undergone endoscopy with an instrument previously used on an infected patient. In addition, the seroconversion rate was lower than that for control populations not undergoing endoscopy.

Transmission of HBV appears to be rare, even with inadequate cleaning and disinfection, and there are no reported cases of transmission when accepted guidelines have been followed. The possible transmission of pathogens to 236 persons exposed to an endoscope processed in a flawed automated endoscope washer/disinfector in a gastrointestinal endoscopy unit was investigated. During a 60-month period, 197 subjects (83.5%) were followed up and no cases of acute hepatitis B, HIV, or HCV infection were observed.[37] A separate prospective study was performed to evaluate HCV and HBV transmission after GI endoscopy, including biopsy. In 17 subjects who were positive for HBsAg and 8 subjects who were positive for anti-HCV antibody, the endoscopes were cleaned on site by suctioning and flushing the air and water channels with an enzyme detergent. First samples were then collected by flushing 5 mL of sterile water through each channel. After mechanical reprocessing, second samples were collected. Real-time polymerase chain reactions for HBV virus DNA and HCV RNA showed that HBV DNA was detected in five of the first samples recovered from the suction/accessory channels of the endoscopes, whereas no contamination was detected after reprocessing. The first samples from one water channel and three air channels were also positive for HBV DNA, but were negative after reprocessing. No HCV RNA was detected in any of the samples. The findings suggest that contamination of HBV is common and proper endoscopy reprocessing is critical to minimize the risk for HBV transmission.[38]

TRANSMISSION OF HEPATITIS C AND HEPATITIS B BETWEEN ENDOSCOPY PERSONNEL AND PATIENTS

Although there are several documented cases of transmission of infection from health care workers to patients, there are no documented cases of transmission of HCV or HBV infection from endoscopy personnel to patients. In contrast, there are several reports of documented viral transmission of infection from patients to health care personnel. Potential modes of transmission may include needle stick injury (for HIV),[39,40] and blood splashes to the conjunctiva (for HCV).[41]

PREVENTION OF THE TRANSMISSION OF HEPATITIS C AND HEPATITIS B DURING GASTROINTESTINAL ENDOSCOPY

Over the course of an endoscopic examination the external surface and internal channels of flexible endoscopes are exposed to body fluids and contaminants. Disinfection of these reusable instruments poses special problems. Given their delicate structure, they cannot be autoclaved. Therefore endoscopy processing should be achieved by proper mechanical cleaning followed by high-level disinfection, rinsing, drying, and storage. Stringent guidelines for the reprocessing of flexible endoscopes were developed by the ASGE and the Society for Health care Epidemiology of America, who convened with representatives from physician, nursing and infection control organizations, industry leaders, and federal and state agencies. This conference resulted in the 2003 multi-society guideline for reprocessing of flexible gastrointestinal endoscopes.[7] Since that time, there have been no reported cases of transmission of infection when these high-level disinfection guidelines have been followed. In the absence of defective equipment, all subsequent reported cases of transmission of infection have resulted from failure to adhere to these guidelines.

General infection control principles should be strictly followed by all endoscopy personnel. Appropriate aseptic techniques and safe injection practices should be followed. The practice of reuse of syringes and use of contaminated multiple-dose drug vials should be avoided and single-use drug vials are recommended. Standard precautions from the Occupational Safety and Health Act (OSHA) should be followed.[42] Endoscopy personnel should be aware of the dangers of blood and other body fluids, contaminated equipment, and the modes of disease transmission. It is prudent to apply standard precautions for blood and body fluids when interacting with all patients. OSHA mandates that all employees should be immunized against HBV.[43] A variety of other measures are needed for optimal infection control among employees, before and during the period of employment. In particular, an effective and readily accessible employee health service plays a critical role in the management of postexposure prophylaxis.[44]

Following the endoscopic procedure, exposed surfaces should be thoroughly cleaned of visible contaminants and then disinfected with a hospital disinfectant registered by the US Environmental Protection Agency.[45] Hand wash is mandatory before and after each patient interaction and each endoscopy procedure, irrespective of whether gloves are used. Isolation precautions in potentially infected patients should be maintained when patients are transported to endoscopy units. Needles should be discarded in sharps containers without recapping to avoid inadvertent sticks. Endoscopy units should adopt needleless systems for administration of parenteral drugs whenever feasible. Endoscopy-unit infection-control policies should address procedure-room work areas, separation of soiled and clean tasks and handling of specimens, tissues, soiled linens, and contaminated wastes.[46]

In summary, HCV and HBV transmission during GI endoscopy can occur, but fortunately is rare. Proper cleaning, disinfection, and reprocessing of endoscopies and accessories, and appropriate administration of intravenous drugs help to minimize the risk for infection transmission.

REFERENCES

1. Available at: http://news.yahoo.com/s/ap/20090326/ap_on_re_us/veterans_colonoscopies. Accessed March 27, 2009.
2. Spach DH, Silverstein FE, Stamm WE. Transmission of infection by gastro-intestinal endoscopy and bronchoscopy. Ann Intern Med 1993;118:117–28.
3. ASGE Standards of Practice Committee. Banerjee S, Shen B, et al. Infection control during GI endoscopy. Gastrointest Endosc 2008;67:781–90.
4. Ponchon T. Transmission of hepatitis C and prion diseases through digestive endoscopy: evaluation of risk and recommended practices. Endoscopy 1997; 29:199–202.
5. Labus B, Sands L, Rowley P, et al. Acute hepatitis C virus infections attributed to unsafe injection practices at an endoscopy clinic—Nevada, 2007. JAMA 2008; 299:2738–40.
6. Cleaning and disinfection of equipment for gastrointestinal flexible endoscopy: interim recommendations of a Working Party of the British Society of Gastroenterology. Gut 1988;29:1134–51.
7. Nelson DB, Jarvis WR, Rutala WA, et al. Multi-society guideline for reprocessing flexible gastrointestinal endoscopes. Gastrointest Endosc 2003;58:1–8.
8. Nelson DB, Muscarella LF. Current issues in endoscope reprocessing and infection control during gastrointestinal endoscopy. World J Gastroenterol 2006;12: 3953–64.
9. Mele A, Spada E, Sagliocca L, et al. Risk of parenterally transmitted hepatitis following exposure to surgery or other invasive procedures: results from the hepatitis surveillance system in Italy. J Hepatol 2001;35:284–9.
10. Hauri AM, Armstrong GL, Hutin YJ. The global burden of disease attributable to contaminated injections given in health care settings. Int J STD AIDS 2004;15: 7–16.
11. Courouce AM, French Blood Transfusion Centers. Seroconversion to HCV in repeat blood donors. Proceedings of IX Triennial International Symposium on viral hepatitis and liver disease, Rome, 21–25 April 1996. In: Rizzetto M, Purcell RH, Gerin JL, et al, editors. Viral hepatitis and liver disease. Torino (Italy): Edizioni Minerva Medica; 1997. p. 250–2.
12. Nelson DB. Infectious disease complications of GI endoscopy: part II, exogenous infections. Gastrointest Endosc 2003;57:695–711.

13. Tennenbaum R, Colardelle P, Chochon M, et al. Hepatitis C after retrograde cholangiography [letter]. Gastroenterol Clin Biol 1993;17:763–4.
14. Bronowicki JP, Venard V, Botte C, et al. Patient-to-patient transmission of hepatitis C virus during colonoscopy. N Engl J Med 1997;337:237–40.
15. Delarocque-Astagneau E, Pillonel J, De Valk H, et al. An incident case-control study of modes of hepatitis C virus transmission in France. Ann Epidemiol 2007;17:755–62.
16. Habib M, Mohamed MK, Abdel-Aziz F, et al. Hepatitis C virus infection in a community in the Nile Delta: risk factors for seropositivity. Hepatology 2001; 33:248–53.
17. Medhat A, Shehata M, Magder LS, et al. Hepatitis C in a community in Upper Egypt: risk factors for infection. Am J Trop Med Hyg 2002;66:33–8.
18. Tawk HM, Vickery K, Bisset L, et al. Infection in Endoscopy Study Group. The significance of transfusion in the past as a risk for current hepatitis B and hepatitis C infection: a study in endoscopy patients. Transfusion 2005;45: 807–13.
19. Nelson DB. What is the risk of transmission of hepatitis C virus during digestive endoscopy? Nat Clin Pract Gastroenterol Hepatol 2005;2:560–1.
20. Chanzy B, Duc-Bin DL, Rousset B, et al. Effectiveness of a manual disinfection procedure in eliminating hepatitis C virus from experimentally contaminated endoscopes. Gastrointest Endosc 1999;50:147–51.
21. Cronmiller JR, Nelson DK, Salman G, et al. Antimicrobial efficacy of endoscopic disinfection procedures: a controlled, multifactorial investigation. Gastrointest Endosc 1999;50:152–8.
22. Petersen BT. Gaining perspective on reprocessing of GI endoscopes [editorial]. Gastrointest Endosc 1999;50:287–91.
23. Ciancio A, Manzini P, Castagno F, et al. Digestive endoscopy is not a major risk factor for transmitting hepatitis C virus. Ann Intern Med 2005;142:903–9.
24. Mikhail NN, Lewis DL, Omar N, et al. Prospective study of cross-infection from upper-GI endoscopy in a hepatitis C-prevalent population. Gastrointest Endosc 2007;65:584–8.
25. Morris IM, Cattle DS, Smits BJ. Letter: endoscopy and transmission of hepatitis B. Lancet 1975;2:1152.
26. Seefeld U, Bansky G, Jaeger M, et al. Prevention of hepatitis B virus transmission by the gastrointestinal fibrescope. Successful disinfection with an aldehyde liquid. Endoscopy 1981;13:238–9.
27. Birnie GG, Quigley EM, Clements GB, et al. Endoscopic transmission of hepatitis B virus. Gut 1983;24:171–4.
28. McDonald GB, Silverstein FE. Can gastrointestinal endoscopy transmit hepatitis B to patients? Gastrointest Endosc 1976;22:168–70.
29. McClelland DB, Burrell CJ, Tonkin RW, et al. Hepatitis B: absence of transmission by gastrointestinal endoscopy. Br Med J 1978;1:23–4.
30. Morgan AG, McAdam WA, Walker BE. Hepatitis B and endoscopy. Br Med J 1978;1:369.
31. Moncada RE, Denes AE, Berquist KR, et al. Inadvertent exposure of endoscopy patients to viral hepatitis B. Gastrointest Endosc 1978;24:231–2.
32. Chiaramonte M, Farini R, Truscia D, et al. Risk of hepatitis B virus infection following upper gastrointestinal endoscopy: a prospective study in an endemic area. Hepatogastroenterology 1983;30:189–91.
33. Hoofnagle JH, Blake J, Buskell-Bales Z, et al. Lack of transmission of type B hepatitis by fiberoptic upper endoscopy. J Clin Gastroenterol 1980;2:65–9.

34. Ayoola EA. The risk of type B hepatitis infection in flexible fiberoptic endoscopy. Gastrointest Endosc 1981;27:60–2.
35. Villa E, Pasquinelli C, Rigo G, et al. Gastrointestinal endoscopy and HBV infection: no evidence for a causal relationship. A prospective controlled study. Gastrointest Endosc 1984;30:15–7.
36. Lok A, Lai C, Hui W, et al. Absence of transmission of hepatitis B by fibreoptic upper gastrointestinal endoscopy. J Gastroenterol Hepatol 1987;2:175–90.
37. Vanhems P, Gayet-Ageron A, Ponchon T, et al. Follow-up and management of patients exposed to a flawed automated endoscope washer-disinfector in a digestive diseases unit. Infect Control Hosp Epidemiol 2006;27:89–92 [Erratum in: 2006;27:431].
38. Ishino Y, Ido K, Sugano K. Contamination with hepatitis B virus DNA in gastrointestinal endoscope channels: risk of infection on reuse after on-site cleaning. Endoscopy 2005;37:548–51.
39. Oksenhendler E, Harzic M, Le Roux JM, et al. HIV infection with seroconversion after a superficial needlestick injury to the finger. N Engl J Med 1986;315:582.
40. Wallace MR, Harrison WO. HIV seroconversion with progressive disease in health care worker after needlestick injury. Lancet 1988;1:1454.
41. Sartori M, La Terra G, Aglietta M, et al. Transmission of hepatitis C via blood splash into conjunctiva. Scand J Infect Dis 1993;25:270–1.
42. Centers for Disease Control. Update: universal precautions for prevention of transmission of human immunodeficiency virus, hepatitis b virus and other blood-borne pathogens in health-care settings. MMWR Morb Mortal Wkly Rep 1988;37: 377–82, 87–8.
43. Centers for Disease Control. Protection against Viral Hepatitis: recommendations of the Immunization Practices Advisory Committee (ACIP). MMWR Morb Mortal Wkly Rep 1990;39:S-2.
44. Diekema DJ, Doebbeling BN. Employee health and infection control. Infect Control Hosp Epidemiol 1995;16:292–301.
45. Rutala WA. APIC guideline for selection and use of disinfectants. 1994, 1995, and 1996 APIC Guidelines Committee. Association for professionals in infection control and epidemiology, Inc [see comment]. Am J Infect Control 1996;24: 313–42.
46. Decker MD. The OSHA bloodborne hazard standard. Infect Control Hosp Epidemiol 1992;13:407–17.

Health Care–Associated Transmission of Hepatitis B and C in Oncology Care

Michael P. Stevens, MD[a],*, Michael B. Edmond, MD, MPH, MPA[a,b]

KEYWORDS

- Health care–associated infections • Hepatitis B
- Hepatitis C • Oncology

Before the identification and routine screening of blood products for hepatitis B (HBV) and hepatitis C (HCV), oncology patients were at particularly high risk of nosocomially acquired infection with these viruses, which was largely related to the high transfusion demands of this population.[1–3] This was especially true for patients with hematologic malignancies, and multiple studies have found an association between blood product administration and acquiring infection with HBV and HCV.[1,4] Following the initiation of screening for hepatitis B surface antigen (HBsAg) in 1972 and surrogate marker screening for non-A, non-B (NANB) hepatitis (which subsequently has been predominantly attributed to hepatitis C) in 1986 and for antibody to hepatitis C in 1990, the incidence of post-transfusion infection secondary to these viruses dropped dramatically.[5–7] Testing for HBV and HCV has since been significantly refined, increasing sensitivity.[6–8] The current risk of developing infection with HBV and HCV is related to receiving blood products donated within the "window phase" of infection for these viruses and the overall prevalence of these infections in the blood donor population.[8–10] As the sensitivity of screening techniques developed and used for HBV and HCV has increased, breaches in infection control have played a more prominent role in the transmission of these viruses in inpatient and outpatient oncology settings.

HEPATITIS B TRANSMISSION RELATED TO BLOOD PRODUCT ADMINISTRATION

Historically, oncology patients have been at high risk of nosocomially acquired infection with HBV, with the risk of transmission being associated with blood product

---

Neither author has any conflicts of interest.

[a] Division of Infectious Diseases, Virginia Commonwealth University Medical Center, 1201 East Marshall Street, P.O. Box 980019, Richmond, Virginia 23298-0019, USA

[b] Epidemiology and Community Health, Virginia Commonwealth University School of Medicine, 1201 East Marshall Street, P.O. Box 980019, Richmond, Virginia 23298-0019, USA

* Corresponding author.

E-mail address: mstevens2@mcvh-vcu.edu (M.P. Stevens).

Clin Liver Dis 14 (2010) 69–74

doi:10.1016/j.cld.2009.11.006

1089-3261/10/$ – see front matter

administration.[1] In the United States, screening for HBsAg was adopted in 1972, with hepatitis B core antibody (anti-HBc) testing being added in 1986.[11] NANB hepatitis was a recognized clinical entity before the identification of HCV (which is now believed to have accounted for most of the cases of NANB hepatitis). Multiple studies of post-transfusion hepatitis indicated an increased risk of infection with NANB hepatitis in association with the transfusion of anti-HBc–positive units, presumably secondary to similar risk factors for HBV and NANB hepatitis acquisition. Based on these data, anti-HBc was added to donor blood screening as a surrogate marker for NANB hepa-titis. However, adding this test to blood donor screening also helped to identify donors who were in the "window phase" of HBV infection (wherein HBsAg has disappeared but antibody to HBsAg is not yet present).[11,12] More recently, nucleic acid testing (NAT) for HBV has been developed.[6,13]

One Polish study of children treated for cancer from 1974 to 2000 noted that 74 of 119 patients (62.2%) had evidence of exposure to HBV before 1992. The proportion of patients infected with HBV decreased to 8 of 168 (4.8%) from 1992 to 1995 and further decreased to 2 of 108 (1.9%) from 1999 to October 2000. The decrease in the propor-tion of patients infected with HBV was attributed to blood product screening, HBV immunization and immunoprophylaxis, educational programs, and improvements in infection control.[1] A study in Turkey, a country where the seroprevalence of HBV is noted to be high, of children with solid tumors treated between 1994 and 1995 found a HBV seropositivity of 4% at time of diagnosis that increased to 20% following cancer treatment, occurring despite blood product screening for HBsAg. The high rate of seroconversion was partly related to the high prevalence of disease in the donor pop-ulation.[14] HBV transmission has also occurred following bone marrow transplantation.[15]

The risk of transfusion-related HBV infection in the United States has been esti-mated at 1 in 205,000 to 1 in 488,000 transfused units.[16] In the United States, a program to eliminate HBV transmission was established in 1991 and involves universal vaccination of children, adolescents, and adults at risk of developing infec-tion with HBV, with more than an 80% decline in the rate of new infections between 1991 and 2006. In 2006, the overall incidence of symptomatic, acute cases of infection with HBV was 1.6 cases per 100,000 people. For the cases who provided epidemio-logic data, 13 of 2048 (0.6%) noted having a blood transfusion in the 6 months before symptom development.[17]

The risks of acquiring infection with HBV during oncology therapy are related to the sensitivity of the testing used for blood product screening and the prevalence of disease in the population.[10,12] There is a great disparity between regions in the prevalence of HBV infection. For example, more than 80% of people in West Africa have evidence of exposure to HBV and less than 0.5%, in the United Kingdom.[6] In countries where less sensitive screening methods are used and the prevalence of HBV is high, the risk of disease acquisition via blood product administration is also relatively high.[10]

HEPATITIS C TRANSMISSION RELATED TO BLOOD PRODUCT ADMINISTRATION

Before the identification of HCV and the development of screening tests for this virus, oncology patients were at particularly high risk of developing infection with this agent. Risk of developing infection has been associated with the volume of blood products administered and is also related to the prevalence of disease in the blood donor pop-ulation.[1,4,10] Screening of donated blood for antibodies against hepatitis C began in the United States in 1990 with an enzyme immunoassay (EIA), which was replaced by a more sensitive EIA in 1992; subsequently more sensitive tests have been developed, including NAT.[6,7,18]

One Italian study looked at stored serum for patients treated for childhood cancer from 1968 to 1982 (before HCV was identified and specific testing existed) and found that 56 of 114 children (49%) were HCV-RNA–positive following treatment.[2] Another Polish study of children treated for cancer from 1974 to 2000 found that 50 of 92 children (54.3%) who had received therapy before HCV blood donation testing became available were seropositive for HCV. In contrast, for 108 patients who were tested between 1999 and 2000, there were only 3 new infections with HCV identified (2.8%).[1] HCV acquisition has also been documented following bone marrow transplantation from HCV-positive donors.[19]

Increasingly more sophisticated tests, including NAT, have decreased the risk of acquiring HCV from a blood transfusion in the United States to 1 in 1.8 million units of blood transfused.[9] In 2006, the rate of acute infections with HCV in the United States was 0.3 cases per 100,000 people. Of the cases providing epidemiologic data, 0 of 318 reported having a blood transfusion in the 6 months before symptom onset.[17] As previously noted for HBV acquisition, the risk of developing HCV from blood product administration is higher in countries using less sensitive detection techniques and with a higher prevalence of disease in the donor population.[10]

TRANSMISSION OF HEPATITIS B AND C RELATED TO BREACHES IN INFECTION CONTROL

As screening techniques for HBV and HCV have become more sophisticated, the risk of acquiring infection with these viruses in the oncology setting has increasingly been related to breaches in infection control.[20] One Italian study of 658 patients who had initiated treatment for childhood cancer before 1990 (the year specific tests became available for blood product screening for HCV) found that 117 (17.8%) had evidence of exposure to HCV. Of these patients, approximately 20% had not received blood products, and the investigators postulate that the development of HCV infection was partially secondary to suboptimal infection control techniques.[21] Another Swedish study described 2 HCV outbreaks that occurred on a pediatric oncology ward in the 1990s, with disease transmission ultimately being attributed to the improper use of multidose vials of saline and heparin.[22] Several other studies of HCV outbreaks on inpatient hematology and oncology wards postulated that virus aerosolization might have been a mechanism of virus transmission, although these same studies also noted the possible use of contaminated multidose vials on these units.[20,23] Later, in 2000 to 2001 an outbreak of HCV occurred in a Nebraska oncology clinic that was associated with using contaminated syringes to draw off saline bags used for multiple patients. More than 600 patients were exposed and 99 were found to be infected with HCV.[24,25]

The adoption of and compliance with optimal infection control practices is critical in preventing the transmission of HBV and HCV in oncology settings. The Centers for Disease Control and Prevention have outlined guidelines for safe injection practices that include never using a single syringe on multiple patients, never entering a communal medication vial with a used needle or syringe, and using dedicated medication vials whenever possible.[26] The adoption of optimal infection control practices is especially important for patients receiving treatment in outpatient clinics, because regulations and oversight in these settings have traditionally been less stringent or absent when compared with inpatient areas.[27,28] Indeed, as oncology care has increasingly moved from inpatient wards to outpatient clinics, the importance of optimizing infection control in these settings has become paramount. Infection control policies should be put into place in all outpatient facilities, single-use syringes should replace multidose vials or communal saline bags, and regular employee education on issues with infection control should occur.[27,28] Nonimmunized health care workers and at-risk patients should be vaccinated for hepatitis B.[17] Additionally, there should be regular oversight of an individual facility's infection control program, and administrators should be empowered to suspend programs deemed unsafe. Unfortunately, the true incidence of disease acquisition that occurs with HBV and HCV in outpatient oncology clinics relating to poor infection control practices is unknown, partly relating to the lack of a dedicated disease surveillance system in this setting. Optimally, a system for disease surveillance and case investigation should be created for outpatient oncology clinics.[27,28]

SUMMARY

The risk of acquiring HBV and HCV in the oncology setting was historically high and predominantly related to blood product administration in the prescreening era.[1–3] With the development of progressively more sophisticated testing for HBV and HCV, breaches in infection control have played an increasingly prominent role in disease transmission.[20] Optimizing infection control in inpatient and outpatient oncology settings is essential to preventing the transmission of HBV and HCV in these settings. In particular, infection control policies should be implemented in all outpatient facilities, single-use syringes should replace multidose vials or communal saline bags, employees and patients at high risk of developing infection with HBV should be immunized, and regular employee education on issues with infection control should occur.[17,27,28] There should also be regular oversight of an individual facility's infection control program, administrators should be empowered to suspend programs deemed unsafe, and a system for disease surveillance and case investigation should be created for use in outpatient oncology clinics.[27,28] As oncology care is increasingly delivered in the outpatient setting, it has become critical that outpatient infection control practices be optimized to decrease the risk of transmitting HBV and HCV.

REFERENCES

1. Styczynski J, Wysocki M, Koltan S, et al. Epidemiologic aspects and preventive strategy of hepatitis B and C viral infections in children with cancer. Pediatr Infect Dis J 2001;20(11):1042–9.
2. Locasciulli A, Testa M, Pontisso P, et al. Prevalence and natural history of hepatitis C infection in patients cured of childhood leukemia. Blood 1997;90(11):4628–33.
3. Locasciulli A, Alberti A. Hepatitis C virus serum markers and liver disease in children with leukemia. Leuk Lymphoma 1995;17(3–4):245–9.
4. Hetherington ML, Buchanan GR. Elevated serum transaminase values during therapy for acute lymphoblastic leukemia correlate with prior blood transfusions. Cancer 1988;62(8):1614–8.
5. Goldfield M, Black HC, Bill J, et al. The consequences of administering blood pretested for HBs Ag by third generation techniques: a progress report. Am J Med Sci 1975;270(2):335–42.
6. Allain JP, Stramer SL, Carneiro-Proietti AB, et al. Transfusion-transmitted infectious diseases. Biologicals 2009;37(2):71–7.
7. Donahue JG, Muñoz A, Ness PM, et al. The declining risk of post-transfusion hepatitis C virus infection. N Engl J Med 1992;327(6):369–73.

8. O'Brien SF, Yi QL, Fan W, et al. Current incidence and estimated residual risk of transfusion-transmitted infections in donations made to Canadian blood services. Transfusion 2007;47(2):316–25.
9. Busch MP, Glynn SA, Stramer SL, et al. A new strategy for estimating risks of transfusion-transmitted viral infections based on rates of detection of recently infected donors. Transfusion 2005;45(2):254–64.
10. Shang G, Seed CR, Wang F, et al. Residual risk of transfusion-transmitted viral infections in Shenzhen, China 2001 through 2004. Transfusion 2007;47(3):529–39.
11. Chambers LA, Popovsky MA. Decrease in reported posttransfusion hepatitis. Contributions of donor screening for alanine aminotransferase and antibodies to hepatitis B core antigen and changes in the general population. Arch Intern Med 1991;151(12):2445–8.
12. Busch MP. Prevention of transmission of hepatitis B, hepatitis C and human immunodeficiency virus infections through blood transfusion by anti-HBc testing. Vox Sang 1998;74(Suppl 2):147–54.
13. Stramer SL. Current risks of transfusion-transmitted agents: a review. Arch Pathol Lab Med 2007;131(5):702–7.
14. Kebudi R, Ayan I, Yílmaz G, et al. Seroprevalence of hepatitis B, hepatitis C and human immunodeficiency virus infections in children with cancer at diagnosis and following therapy in Turkey. Med Pediatr Oncol 2000;34(2):102–5.
15. Locasciulli A, Nava S, Sparano P, et al. Infections with hepatotropic viruses in children treated with allogeneic bone marrow transplantation. Bone Marrow Transplant 1998;21(Suppl 2):S75–7.
16. Dodd RY, Notari EP, Stramer SL. Current prevalence and incidence of infectious disease markers and estimated window-period risk in the American Red Cross blood donor population. Transfusion 2002;42(8):975–9.
17. Wasley A, Grytdal S, Gallagher K. Surveillance for acute viral hepatitis-United States, 2006. MMWR Surveill Summ 2008;57(2):1–24.
18. Gretch DR. Diagnostic tests for hepatitis C. Hepatology 1997;26(3 Suppl 1):43S–7S.
19. Shuhart MC, Myerson D, Childs BH, et al. Marrow transplantation from hepatitis C virus seropositive donors: transmission rate and clinical course. Blood 1994; 84(9):3229–35.
20. Silini E, Locasciulli A, Santoleri L, et al. Hepatitis C virus infection in a hematology ward: evidence of nosocomial transmission and impact on hematologic disease outcome. Haematologica 2002;87(11):1200–8.
21. Cesaro S, Petris MG, Rossetti F, et al. Chronic hepatitis C virus infection after treatment for pediatric malignancy. Blood 1997;90(3):1315–20.
22. Widell A, Christensson B, Wiebe T, et al. Epidemiologic and molecular investigation of outbreaks of hepatitis C virus infection on a pediatric oncology service. Ann Intern Med 1999;130(2):130–4.
23. Allander T, Gruber A, Naghavi M, et al. Frequent patient-to-patient transmission of hepatitis C virus in a haematology ward. Lancet 1995;345(8950):603–7.
24. Centers for Disease Control and Prevention (CDC). Transmission of hepatitis B and C viruses in outpatient settings-New York, Oklahoma and Nebraska, 2000-2002. MMWR Morb Mortal Wkly Rep 2003;52(38):901–6.
25. Macedo de Oliveira A, White KL, Leschinsky DP, et al. An outbreak of hepatitis C virus infections among outpatients at a hematology/oncology clinic. Ann Intern Med 2005;142(11):898–902.
26. Centers for Disease Control and Prevention. Injection safety information for providers. Available at: http://www.cdc.gov/ncidod/dhqp/ps_providerInfo.html. Accessed June 17, 2009.

27. Wenzel RP, Edmond MB. Patient-to-patient transmission of hepatitis C virus. Ann Intern Med 2005;142(11):940–1.

28. Thompson ND, Perz JF, Moorman AC, et al. Nonhospital health care-associated hepatitis B and C virus transmission: United States 1998-2008. Ann Intern Med 2009;150(1):33–9.

Management of Acute Hepatitis B

Mitchell L. Shiffman, MD

KEYWORDS

• Hepatitis B virus • Acute HBV • Chronic HBV • HBV vaccine

Hepatitis B virus (HBV) infection is the most common cause of chronic liver disease worldwide. It is currently estimated that over 350 million persons have chronic HBV.[1] These individuals serve as the source for acute infection in susceptible individuals. The prevalence of the chronic HBV reservoir varies significantly by race, ethnicity, and geography of birth. This variation has been reviewed previously[2] and by Jensen in this issue of *Clinics in Liver Disease*. In those areas of the world with the highest prevalence for HBV (Southeast Asia, China, the Korean peninsula, sub-Saharan Africa, and many Caribbean Islands) 70% to 90% of the population has serologic markers of past or current infection. In contrast, less than 2% of the population of North America and most European nations have been exposed to HBV. In these low-prevalence areas of the world nearly half of all persons with HBV are immigrants from areas of the world with high prevalence, or are the first-generation offspring of persons who immigrated from high-prevalence areas. In North America, approximately half of all persons with chronic HBV are of Asian descent.[3]

Acute hepatitis B infection occurs when an "at risk" individual becomes infected with the HBV. In areas of the world with high prevalence for HBV the vast majority of all new infections are the result of vertical transmission to newborns from their mothers, or from horizontal transmission from family members to young children or adolescents within the home.[1] In areas of the world with low prevalence, acute infection most commonly occurs in nonvaccinated teenagers or adults who have sexual interactions, share items of personal hygiene, or objects to administer illicit drugs with a chronically infected person. In the vast majority of these cases, the patient is unaware their partner in these activities has chronic HBV. Patients can also acquire HBV during medical procedures, either through breaks in universal precautions from health care workers with chronic HBV or from contaminated medical equipment. These issues are discussed by Shen, Edmonds, and Younai in their articles elsewhere in this issue. Although serologic testing has been utilized to screen blood products for

Dr Shiffman has been a consultant and speaker for Roche laboratories and Gilead Pharmaceuticals, and has received clinical research funding for studies in patients with chronic HBV from Hofmann-LaRoche, Gilead, Bristol-Myers-Squib, and Pharamcet.
Bon Secours Health System, Liver Institute of Virginia, Richmond, VA, USA
E-mail address: mlshiffman@gmail.com

the presence of HBV for several decades, the risk of developing acute HBV following a blood transfusion is currently estimated to occur in 1:63,000 (95% confidence interval: 31,000–147,000) units transfused.[4]

This article reviews the sequence of events and various scenarios that may occur when a susceptible individual becomes infected with HBV. In some cases, persons with chronic HBV can present with jaundice and mimic an acute infection. The management of patients with acute infection, those variants that clinically resemble acute HBV, and strategies to prevent acute infection in susceptible individuals are also discussed.

INCIDENCE AND RISK FACTORS ASSOCIATED WITH ACUTE HBV

The incidence of acute HBV has declined dramatically in nearly all countries since 1992 when the World Health Organization recommended that hepatitis B vaccine be included in all infant immunization programs. Unfortunately, many countries throughout the world, including some in high endemic areas, have failed to adopt this policy. In the United States, the annual incidence of acute HBV declined 78% during the past 2 decades from approximately 232,000 to 51,000 cases annually.[5] This improvement was largely due to the vaccination of persons at risk in the work place, the use of universal precautions for all health care workers, the universal screening of all women during pregnancy, and vaccination of all newborns to mothers with markers of HBV infection. This latter practice has virtually abolished vertical transmission of HBV in the United States and many other developed countries. In 1995 universal vaccination of adolescents was implemented in the United States. Unfortunately, this practice has done little to reduce the incidence of acute HBV. One of the reasons for this may have been the event that triggered the vaccination of an adolescent; entry to College or University. Strategies to identify and vaccinate those who do not seek higher education and adults who practice high-risk behaviors have been difficult to implement on a national scale. Unfortunately, many primary care providers do not routinely inquire about risk behaviors for communicable diseases, ask about prior vaccination for viral hepatitis B, or administer vaccine when they see patients for routine health maintenance examinations.[6,7] As a result, many adults remain at risk to develop acute HBV.

HBV is transmitted by percutaneous or mucosal exposure through infectious blood or body fluids. Although HBV has been detected in many body fluids, only blood saliva and semen appear to contain sufficient levels of virus to be infectious.[8] The risk of transmitting HBV is directly related to the level of HBV DNA in serum; and this is much greater in patients who are E-antigen positive in serum.[9] HBV remains viable outside the body for more than 7 days, and infection can be acquired if a break in the skin comes in contact with a contaminated environmental surface.[10]

The highest incidence of acute HBV occurs in persons between the ages of 25 and 44 years, and the most common modes of exposure are through sexual activity and intravenous drug use. Heterosexual activity remains the single most common route by which adults transmit HBV. In the United States, this accounts for 39% of all acute infections.[11] The partners or spouses of patients who develop acute HBV are found to have chronic HBV in 20% to 60% of these cases.[12,13] Men who have sex with men account for 24% of cases[14] and intravenous drug use 16% of all acute HBV infections.[15] African Americans represent the racial ethnic group with the highest incidence for acute infection in the United States.[5] Other groups at risk for acute HBV include the nonsexual household contacts of persons with chronic HBV infection[16] and developmentally disabled persons living in long-term care facilities.[17] Such patients are exposed through percutaneous or mucosal exposure to blood and body fluids. Travelers to regions of the world where HBV is endemic may be exposed from intimate contact or prolonged nonintimate interactions with local residents.[18] Patients receiving hemodialysis who have not been previously vaccinated, or have not responded to vaccine are at increased risk for developing acute HBV through breaks in universal precautions.[19] In contrast, first responders such as police and fire officials have similar or lower rates of acute HBV when compared with the general population,[20] and health care workers have the lowest rates of acute HBV because of universal vaccination.[21]

THE CLINICAL SEQUENCE OF ACUTE HBV INFECTION

Following exposure, HBV enters the bloodstream and circulates to the liver. Although the precise mechanism by which HBV enters hepatocytes and other cells remains undefined, recent studies have suggested that binding of the HBV pre-S protein to an asialoglycoprotein receptor on the cell surface of hepatocytes is essential for viral entry.[22] In contrast, the S-protein does not seem to be essential for HBV to enter cells; and mutations of the S-gene do not affect the ability of HBV to infect susceptible individuals.[23]

Once infection with HBV has occurred, patients enter an incubation period. During this time patients remain asymptomatic and are typically unaware they have been exposed to HBV. Liver transaminases remain normal. Although factors that affect the duration of the incubation period remain obscure, this is likely dependent on the size of the HBV inoculum, the ability of cell surface receptors to capture HBV, and the immune response to acute HBV infection.[24] Variations in host genetics no doubt affect each of these interactions. Once HBV has entered the hepatocyte it begins to replicate, HBV proteins are expressed on the hepatocyte cell surface, an immune response is initiated against infected hepatocytes, liver cells are injured, and the serum level of HBV DNA begins to rise. The incubation period from infection to the time liver transaminases first become elevated may last from 1 to 6 months, with an average duration of 60 days.[25,26]

The prodrome, or clinical presentation, of acute HBV infection varies widely depending on the age and the immune status of the patient. Infants, children younger than 5 years, and immunosuppressed adults are in most cases completely asymptomatic. Acute HBV infection is often unrecognized in these individuals. In the majority of patients the symptoms of acute HBV infection are nonspecific, insidious, and short-lived. The most common symptoms include anorexia, malaise, nausea, vomiting, and abdominal pain, and these may last for only 1 to 5 days.[27] If these symptoms are mild, if the patient does not seek medical attention, or if liver transaminases are not tested during a medical evaluation for these symptoms, the diagnosis of acute HBV infection could easily be missed. Such individuals may be found years later to have serologic evidence of prior exposure to HBV or chronic disease.

The icteric phase of acute HBV infection occurs with the onset of jaundice. However, only about 30% of all patients with acute HBV develop jaundice. The average time from infection to the onset of jaundice, when this occurs, is 90 days.[25,26] It is the appearance of icteric sclera, not the nonspecific symptoms of the prodrome, that leads the vast majority of patients with acute HBV to seek medical attention. The age at which the patient becomes infected is directly related to the likelihood they will develop acute icteric HBV and the severity of the acute event (**Fig. 1**). Approximately 30% to 50% of teenagers and adults with acute HBV develop jaundice.

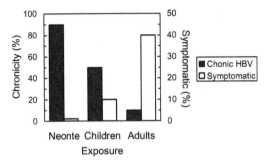

Fig. 1. Relationship between the development of symptomatic acute icteric hepatitis, age and the likelihood of developing chronic HBV.

In contrast, jaundice rarely occurs in infants and young children.[27] Jaundice may be mild or pronounced, and this is dependent on the severity of the host immune response directed against HBV. When jaundice does occur, it may last for as little as 1 to 2 days if mild, or for as long as several weeks if pronounced.

The final phase of acute HBV infection is resolution. This phase is associated with a decline in liver transaminases back to within the limits of normal and resolution of all symptoms. In general, liver transaminases will normalize within 2 to 8 weeks following the acute event. However, the rate at which the symptoms of acute HBV resolve varies considerably. The rate is primarily dependent on the severity of symptoms during the acute event. For those patients with mild acute HBV and who were minimally symptomatic resolution may occur rapidly, within just a few days of the onset of these mild nonspecific symptoms. In contrast, patients with acute icteric HBV, particularly those with a serum bilirubin greater than 10 mg/dL, will typically experience severe fatigue and nausea for weeks to months before jaundice and resolution of fatigue is complete. Resolution of acute HBV is also associated with elimination of virus from the blood and the appearance of anti-HB surface (anti-HBs), which confers long-lasting immunity from reinfection (**Fig. 2**).

Resolution of HBV with development of protective anti-HBs is directly related to the patient's age at the time of infection and the severity of the clinical presentation (see **Fig. 1**). When teenagers and adults develop acute HBV infection they are often symptomatic and jaundiced. Nearly all such patients develop complete resolution of the acute infection with development of protective anti-HBs. In contrast, the development

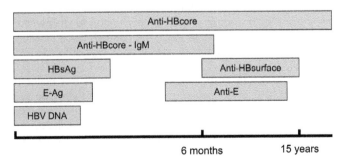

Fig. 2. Appearance and disappearance of HBV antigens and antibodies in response to acute HBV infection.

of chronic HBV following acute infection in teenagers and adults is almost exclusively limited to those patients who were relatively asymptomatic and did not develop jaundice during the acute event.[27] Many of these patients are unaware they were exposed to HBV and are found to have chronic disease years later. Children younger than 5 years are rarely symptomatic or jaundiced following exposure to HBV. Nearly 95% of these children and infants fail to resolve this infection and develop chronic HBV.

SEROLOGIC MARKERS OF HBV INFECTION

Proteins (antigens) produced by HBV and antibodies produced by the host immune response against certain HBV antigens can be measured and utilized to determine the clinical phase of HBV infection. The appearance and disappearance of these antigens and antibodies following acute infection is depicted in **Fig. 2**. HB surface antigen (HBsAg) appears in serum during the incubation phase, approximately 2 to 6 weeks before the onset of symptoms.[25,26] Highly sensitive molecular virologic assays can detect HBV DNA in the serum of persons during the incubation phase, approximately 10 to 20 days before the appearance of HBsAg.[28] This finding has led some clinicians to advocate virologic testing for blood bank screening. Recent studies have suggested that screening blood products in the United States with nucleic acid tests could prevent 30 to 35 cases of acute post-transfusion HBV. However, the majority of these patients would resolve the acute HBV infection, and virologic testing for HBV on donated blood would cost the health care industry an additional $39 to 130 million annually.[29]

Anti-HB core (anti-HBc) appears at the onset of symptoms or with liver test abnormalities. Hepatitis B core antigen is produced intracellularly and can be detected by immunohistochemical staining of liver histologic specimens in patients with acute or chronic infection. Core antigen does not gain access to the serum in any appreciable amounts and is not routinely measured.[25,26] During acute infection the host immune response produces both IgG and IgM antibodies against HBV core. Detection of HBsAg along with anti-HBc IgM is the serologic hallmark of acute HBV infection.[30] Both of these serologic markers remain detectable during the prodrome and icteric phases of an acute HBV infection. As patients enter the resolution phase, HBsAg is lost but anti-HBs does not appear for many weeks to months.[25,26,28] During this time, referred to as the window, anti-HBc IgM remains detectable, and this is often the only clue of recent HBV exposure (see **Fig. 2**). HBc IgM remains detectable for approximately 6 months following the acute exposure. Thereafter, IgM antibody is lost. IgG anti-HBc remains detectable lifelong. Patients with acute HBV should be considered infectious and capable of passing HBV to other persons at risk until they develop anti-HBs. Patients with complete resolution of HBV infection have both anti-HBc and anti-HBs. Over many decades following acute HBV infection, the level of anti-HBs may decline to levels that are undetectable with current assays. These patients remain anti-HBc positive as their only marker of previous exposure to HBV.

Other serologic markers produced during acute HBV infection include E-antigen and anti-E. E-antigen is the protein produced by the precore gene, and this appears in serum shortly after HBsAg.[25,26] Thus, E-antigen may appear during the incubation phase and is almost always present during the prodrome. During the resolution phase E-antigen is lost prior to HBsAg and anti-E appears before anti-HBs (see **Fig. 2**). In the vast majority of patients with acute HBV it is not necessary to assay for E-antigen and anti-E; and knowledge of these serologic markers does not aid in the management of the acute infection, alter treatment, or provide prognosis.

An alteration in the genetic sequence of the precore protein is one of the most common mutations of HBV.[31] This mutation produces a stop codon in the precore gene and therefore patients infected with this form of HBV do not express E-antigen. The E-negative strain seems to be more frequently found in persons who were exposed to HBV while in the Mediterranean region and in Asians.[32] If an at-risk person acquires HBV from a patient with E-antigen negative chronic HBV, they will not express E-antigen during the acute phase of the disease or develop anti-E with resolution. Patients who develop acute HBV with an E-negative strain have a very high rate of developing chronic disease, because the E-protein is an important target for the host immune response.[33]

Approximately 27% of persons appear to be coinfected with both wild-type and E-negative strains of HBV.[34] Patients who develop acute HBV following exposure to such patients will be positive for E-antigen and appear to have HBV with "wild-type" virus; the coexistent E-negative strain would only be detectable by nucleic acid mutation testing.[35] Spontaneous resolution of the E-positive "wild-type" virus following an episode of acute HBV will result in the appearance of anti-E. However, the patient will subsequently develop chronic HBV with serologic (HBsAg), biochemical (elevated serum alanine aminotransferase), and virologic (HBV DNA positive) evidence of chronic HBV, as depicted in **Fig. 3**.

IMMUNE MECHANISMS INVOLVED IN RESOLUTION OF ACUTE HBV

Resolution of acute HBV is based on the patient eliciting an effective immune response, and this requires both an innate and adaptive response. The innate immune response controls the initial phase of HBV infection, and results from the production of multiple cytokines by natural killer (NK) cells and Kupffer cells, and production of interferon by infected hepatocytes.[36] Interferon directly inhibits viral replication and viral protein synthesis.[37] Other cytokines cause both antigen-specific and nonspecific T cells to migrate to the liver and then activate these immune cells. The activation of NK cells and cytotoxic CD4 and CD8 lymphocytes is associated with a vigorous, polyclonal response to multiple HBV proteins.[38] The innate response to acute HBV

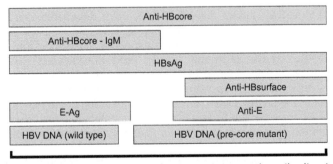

Fig. 3. Appearance and disappearance of HBV antigens and antibodies in a patient coinfected with "wild-type" HBV and an HBV strain with a precore mutation. HBV DNA becomes transiently undetectable as infection with wild-type virus resolves with seroconversion, loss of E-antigen, and appearance of anti-E. The precore mutant strain of HBV is at low levels when coexistent with wild-type virus, but begins to replicate unopposed soon after wild-type virus is cleared.

infection and the recruitment of immune cells into the liver begins during the incuba-tion phase when the patient is still asymptomatic.[38,39]

Over time increasing numbers of NK cells, T lymphocytes, macrophages, and neutrophils are attracted to the liver. Many of these cells produce additional cytokines, and this cyclic process leads to an exponential increase in the number of immune cells invading the liver. The recruitment of these inflammatory cells into the liver results in the histologic finding of hepatic inflammation, the increase in serum liver transami-nases, and the systemic symptoms associated with the prodrome of acute HBV. Eventually this may lead to jaundice.[36]

If this exponential cascade continued, all patients with acute HBV would eventually develop fulminant hepatic failure. Fortunately, nearly all patients down-regulate the immune response to acute HBV. This reduction in the immune response seems to be influenced by a decline in the expression of HBV-specific antigens on the cell surface of hepatocytes and HBc antigen in particular.[40] Resolution of acute HBV is associated with the appearance of anti-HBs and a decline in the number of HBV-specific T cells.[41] However, the responsiveness of these cells to various HBV antigens remains intact, and very high, for decades.[42] Reexposure to HBV in these patients is associated with an appropriate immune response and lack of any clinically significant disease. The presence of HBV DNA in CD8 T cells seems to contribute to this immune responsiveness,[43] suggesting that vial persistence remains in all patients with prior exposure to HBV despite the disappearance of HBV DNA from serum and the pres-ence of anti-HBs.[44]

VARIANTS OF ACUTE HBV INFECTION

The classic adult presentation of acute HBV involves 4 phases as described earlier; the incubation, prodrome, icteric, and resolution phases. However, many patients with acute HBV do not progress through these 4 phases but instead fall into one of the following variant presentations.

Anicteric Acute HBV

Anicteric HBV is the most common variant of acute HBV infection. This presentation is associated with a much higher rate of developing chronic HBV compared with patients who become jaundiced following acute infection (see **Fig. 1**). Unfortunately, the risk of an adult developing chronic HBV following an episode of acute anicteric hepatitis remains undefined because the majority of these patients never come to medical attention. However, it is exceptionally rare for an adult who develops acute icteric HBV to develop chronic HBV.[27] The vast majority of patients with chronic HBV report no history of ever having an episode of acute icteric hepatitis, and only discover they were exposed to HBV years later when found to have serologic markers of previous HBV exposure or chronic disease.

Because the severity of the acute infection is primarily dependent on the host immune response directed against HBV, anicteric acute HBV is commonly observed in immune compromised patients, including persons with human immune deficiency virus (HIV), patients with chronic renal failure on dialysis, and those with diabetes mellitus.[45]

Acute Liver Failure

Acute liver failure (ALF) is defined by the sudden loss of liver function in a patient without preexisting liver disease.[46] About 1% of patients with acute HBV develop ALF. Although precise data are not available, the risk of ALF is much higher, approaching 20%, in patients with acute HBV and hepatitis D virus (HDV) coinfection.[47] The risk of developing ALF with an acute HBV infection is also increased in older individuals and in patients with chronic hepatitis C virus.[48,49]

ALF secondary to acute HBV or HBV plus HDV coinfection is characterized by a marked elevation in serum liver transaminases to values of 1000 IU/L or greater, profound jaundice, coagulopathy, and hepatic encephalopathy. Patients with HDV coinfection appear to improve initially with a decline in serum liver transaminases, but then develop a rebound with a second peak of marked liver transaminase elevations before developing liver failure.[50] It is therefore imperative that patients at risk for HBV plus HDV coinfection be tested for HDV and, if positive, be carefully monitored to ensure that ALF is recognized as soon as possible.

Toxicity from medications, particularly acetaminophen, accounts for over half of all ALF cases in the United States.[46] However, acute HBV infection represents the second most commonly defined etiology for ALF, accounting for 5% to 10% cases. The mean duration from the onset of jaundice to stage III to IV hepatic encephalopathy, elevated intracranial pressure, and brainstem herniation is 6 days. Survival without liver transplantation occurs in only about 25% of patients with ALF secondary to acute HBV. It is therefore imperative that patients with severe acute HBV be transferred to a liver transplant center for evaluation, management, and consideration for liver transplantation if indicated and appropriate.

EXACERBATIONS IN CHRONIC HBV MIMICKING ACUTE INFECTION

Patients with chronic HBV may develop a flare in their disease associated with a marked elevation in serum liver transaminases and jaundice. In some cases hepatic decompensation mimicking ALF may also occur. It is important to recognize and differentiate a flare in a patient with chronic HBV from acute HBV infection.

Spontaneous or Interferon Induced Seroconversion

The majority of patients with E-antigen positive chronic active HBV have slowly progressive liver injury but are generally asymptomatic until they develop advanced cirrhosis or hepatocellular carcinoma. At any time during the clinical course of chronic HBV, patients may develop spontaneous seroconversion with loss of E-antigen and appearance of anti-E. Spontaneous seroconversion occurs in about 5% to 10% of patients with E-antigen positive chronic HBV annually.[51] Although the biologic factors that precipitate spontaneous seroconversion remain obscure, those clinical factors associated with this process include older age and mild to modest elevations in serum aminotransferases.[52] The sequence of events leading to seroconversion is initiated by a sudden decline in the serum HBV DNA level, followed by a marked elevation in serum liver transaminases that then declines to within the limits of normal, loss of E-antigen, and finally the appearance of anti-E. The net result is the conversion from active E-antigen positive chronic HBV to a state of inactive HBV with normal serum liver transaminases and low serum levels of HBV DNA. Although the increase in serum liver transaminases during the flare is usually modest, less than 10 times the upper limit of normal, some patients may develop more pronounced elevations in serum liver transaminases, symptoms of acute hepatitis, and become jaundiced. Serologic evaluation at the time of the flare will typically demonstrate evidence of chronic disease; the presence of HBsAg, anti-HBc, and anti-E. However, in some cases the flare may also be associated with the reappearance of anti-HBc IgM and when this occurs, the patient may be misdiagnosed as having acute HBV rather than chronic HBV with recent seroconversion.[53]

Spontaneous seroconversion is generally a good event in the life cycle of chronic HBV. However, if the patient is older, has had decades of chronic active HBV, and has already developed cirrhosis, the flare associated with spontaneous seroconversion may precipitate hepatic decompensation and liver failure.[54] It is therefore critical to differentiate acute HBV from chronic HBV with seroconversion. Patients with cirrhosis who develop seroconversion frequently have physical and laboratory findings suggestive of cirrhosis, which may include spider angiomata, ascites, edema, and thrombocytopenia.

A flare in serum liver transaminases may also occur when seroconversion occurs in response to treatment with interferon or peginterferon.[55] As in spontaneous seroconversion this is also associated with loss of E-antigen, appearance of anti-E, a marked decline in serum HBV DNA and, over time, a marked improvement in liver histology. Anti-HBc IgM has also been reported to reappear during an interferon-induced flare. Patients with cirrhosis are at increased risk of developing hepatic decompensation if they develop a flare while being treated with interferon or peginterferon. As a result, the treatment of choice for most patients with chronic E-antigen positive HBV and cirrhosis is one the many oral antiviral agents approved for the treatment of chronic HBV.[56]

Cancer Chemotherapy

Reactivation of inactive chronic HBV can occur when these patients receive cancer chemotherapy,[57,58] corticosteroids,[59,60] antitumor necrosis factors,[60,61] methotrexate,[62] or immune suppression following organ transplantation.[63] In each of these scenarios suppression of the immune response leads to a marked increase in HBV replication and the level of HBV DNA in serum, and a flare in serum liver transaminases resembling acute hepatitis. In severe cases patients may develop jaundice and hepatic decompensation. Several studies have demonstrated that prophylactic treatment with either a nucleotide or nucleoside analogue can inhibit HBV replication and prevent the flare in liver transaminases, hepatic decompensation, and death in at-risk patients.[58] It is therefore important that patients, particularly those at risk for chronic HBV infection based on their ethnicity and prior risk factors, be screened for evidence of HBV before the initiation of cancer chemotherapy or before receiving immune suppressive medications. Additional issues related to HBV infection in patients undergoing cancer chemotherapy are discussed elsewhere in this issue by Edmond.

Superinfection with Hepatitis D Virus

HDV is a satellite virus, which cannot exist or be spread in the absence of HBV.[64] The HDV RNA genome is carried within the HBV envelope protein. HDV is most commonly observed in persons who reside along the Mediterranean coast and the northern parts of South America. In the United States, HDV and HBV coinfection is almost exclusively observed in intravenous drug users. The prevalence of HDV has declined significantly throughout the world since 1990.

Patients with chronic HBV who continue to participate in risk behaviors can develop acute HDV superinfection. Acute HDV in these patients is typically associated with severe hepatitis and jaundice.[65] If not previously known to have chronic HBV the patient may be misdiagnosed with acute HBV. Patients with acute HDV superinfection are serologically positive for HBsAg and anti-HBc. The absence of anti-HBc IgM suggests that the patient has chronic HBV and that the acute icteric event is precipitated by another insult. Testing for anti-HDV and HDV RNA will be positive in these patients.

TREATMENT OF ACUTE HBV

The most important treatment for acute HBV is prevention of the primary infection, which is readily accomplished through vaccination. Two types of vaccines against HBV are available; active vaccine and passive immune prophylaxis.

Active Vaccination

Several types of recombinant HBV vaccines are available. Three of these preparations provide immunization against more than one viral or bacterial agent, and are recommended for use in children (**Table 1**). All of these vaccines contain HBsAg produced by yeast into which the HBV surface gene has been inserted. All are administered either subcutaneously or intramuscularly in 3 separate doses over a period of 6 months. All are highly effective in producing a sustained antibody response. High serum titers of anti-HBs develop in more than 95% of vaccinated persons.[66,67] Coexistent administration of peginterferon and ribavirin for treatment of chronic hepatitis C virus (HCV) infection does not seem to alter the response to vaccination.[68] Response to vaccination is less than 75% in persons with chronic HCV infection and is even lower in patients with cirrhosis.[68,69] Patients with chronic renal failure on hemodialysis and HIV also have a suboptimal response to vaccination.[70,71]

Hepatitis B vaccine is extremely effective in preventing vertical and household transmission. The initiation of universal vaccination of newborns in 1984 was associated with a marked decline in the prevalence of chronic HBV in Taiwanese children from 10% to only 0.7% within 15 years.[72,73] In 1991 the American Council on Immunization practices proposed universal vaccination for all newborns and adolescents in

Table 1
Vaccine preparations currently available for HBV

Preparation and Patient Population	Dose Administered	Frequency of Dosing
Recombivax HB		
Children (birth to age 19 y)	5 μg in 0.5 mL	At birth and then 1 and 6 mo after birth
Adolescents (11–15 y)	10 μg in 1.0 mL	0 and in 4–6 mo
Healthy adult (≥20 y)	10 μg in 1.0 mL	0, 1, and 6 mo
Dialysis formulation for dialysis and immunocompromised patients	40 μg in 1.0 mL	0, 1, and 6 mo
Energix-B		
Children (birth to 19 y)	10 μg in 0.5 mL	At birth and then 1 and 6 mo after birth
Healthy adult (≥20 y)	20 μg in 1.0 mL	0, 1, and 6 mo
For dialysis and immunocompromised patients	40 μg—administer 2 1-mL (20 μg) injections	0, 1, 2, and 6 mo
Twinrix (contains hepatitis A virus and HBV)		
Healthy adult (≥18 y)	20 μg in 1.0 mL	0, 1, and 6 mo
Comvax (contains HBV and *Haemophilus influenzae* type b)		
Only to be utilized in children	5 μg in 0.5 mL	2, 4, and 12–15 mo after birth
Pediarix (HBV, diphtheria, tetanus, pertussis and polio viruses)		
Only to be utilized in children	0.5 μg in 0.5 mL	2, 4, 6 mo after birth

the United States. This program has contributed to the dramatic decline in acute HBV observed during the past 2 decades, and has the potential to virtually eliminate HBV within the next several generations.

At the present time it is unclear if booster therapy is necessary in teenagers or adults who received the full course of 3 vaccinations within 6 months as a newborn or young child. In one study, no children living in an endemic area developed HBV even though the titer of anti-HBs declined to undetectable levels in nearly half of these children within 15 years after vaccination.[74] In contrast, another study has demonstrated that about 2% of children living in a highly endemic area for HBV can develop HBsAg if anti-HBs falls below the level of detection following vaccination.[75] However, the majority of children who acquired HBV in this study may not have received the full course of 3 vaccinations. Adults with high-risk sexual behavior who respond to HBV vaccine and achieve anti-HBs levels of more than 10 mIU/mL have been shown to be protected against infection even when the serum level of anti-HBs declines below the level of detection and is undetectable at the time of an exposure.[76,77] As a result, persons who are known to have responded to HBV vaccine do not require booster therapy at any time in the future. In contrast, vaccinated persons without a docu-mented response to vaccination and undetectable anti-HBs at the time of an exposure should probably receive a single booster. Anti-HBs should then be measured 1 month after the booster to assure a response has occurred. If so, no further vaccination is required in the future regardless of anti-HBs titer.

Passive Vaccination with Human Hepatitis B Immune Globulin

Hepatitis B immune globulin (HBIG) is prepared from individuals who were previously exposed to HBV and have high levels of anti-HBs in serum. The serum of these indi-viduals is extensively purified and tested to ensure that no communicable viral disease is present in this preparation.[78] Patients who were recently exposed to a person with chronic HBV and are in the incubation period should receive HBIG. Active vaccine should also be administered to any patient not previously vaccinated. In patients who failed to respond to vaccination the administration of HBIG is the only form of protection when exposed to HBV.

HBIG is administered intramuscularly and provides high serum levels of anti-HBs. In patients who were not truly exposed to HBV, the serum titer of anti-HBs gradually declines following administration of HBIG and becomes undetectable after several months. In patients who were truly exposed to HBV, the high titer of anti-HBs binds circulating virus and converts the exposure into a mild or asymptomatic infection. The vast majority of these patients develop an effective host response against HBV, anti-HBs and long-lasting immunity.

Conservative Management

Adults who develop acute HBV, particularly those who develop symptoms and become jaundiced, almost always resolve the acute infection spontaneously and develop protective anti-HBs. If the systemic symptoms of the acute event, primarily nausea and vomiting, are particularly severe, hospitalization may be required. Antiviral therapy has not been shown to affect the natural history of acute HBV and is not indi-cated. As symptoms resolve, these patients may return to work. It is essential that patients with acute HBV are monitored to ensure they do not develop ALF or chronic HBV. These patients should also be counseled regarding the risk of transmission to sexual and household contacts. These individuals should avoid unprotected sexual activity until they develop anti-HBs, and it is important to remind the patient that this may take up to 6 months.

One of the most important aspects of caring for the patient with acute HBV is to help identify the index patient and the source of the acute infection. This individual is likely unaware he or she has chronic HBV, and informing them of this allows them to seek medical evaluation and treatment. When discussing these issues with the patient it is important they understand that the duration of the prodrome, the time from exposure to the appearance of symptoms, may last up to 6 months. As a result, any individual with whom the patient has had shared risk behaviors within this time period is a possible HBV carrier or could have been exposed to HBV from the patient. The patient should be encouraged to inform these persons that they are at increased risk of having HBV and to seek medical advice.

Use of Oral Anti-HBV Agents in Patients with Acute Liver Failure

Several effective oral agents are currently available for the treatment of chronic HBV.[56] However, because the vast majority of patients with icteric symptomatic acute HBV resolve this infection spontaneously, treatment with one of these nucleotide or nucleoside analogues is not indicated. In addition, it is theoretically possible that treatment of acute HBV with one of these agents could actually increase the risk of developing chronic disease by lowering the serum titer of virus and blunting the immune response.

Lamivudine has been utilized in patients with severe acute HBV associated with high serum levels of aminotransferases, profound jaundice, hepatic encephalopathy, and other features of impending ALF.[79,80] In these reports the majority of patients with these clinical features resolved the severe acute HBV infection without developing ALF and without developing chronic HBV. As a result, it therefore seems reasonable to treat severe HBV with lamivudine or one of the many other oral anti-HBV nucleotide or nucleoside inhibitors when there is high concern for developing ALF.

Reducing the Risk of Vertical Transmission in High-Risk Mothers

Infants remain at risk of acquiring HBV at birth if their mothers are E-antigen positive and have a serum HBV DNA level of more than 10^7 IU/mL.[81,82] Approximately 25% to 40% of infants born to these mothers develop chronic HBV despite receiving HBIG and vaccine. In contrast, infants born to mothers who are E-antigen negative or have a serum HBV DNA level below this critical value do not develop HBV if administered HBIG and vaccine at birth. A double-blind placebo-controlled trial has demonstrated that vertical transmission is significantly reduced when lamivudine is administered to the mother during the third trimester along with HBIG and vaccine to the infant at birth compared with HBIG and vaccine alone.[83] In this study 98% of women treated with lamivudine had a decline in the serum HBV DNA level to less than 1000 IU/mL by the time of delivery. At 1 year of age, 18% of children born to mothers who received lamivudine had developed chronic HBV compared with 39% of placebo-treated mothers. In addition, 84% of the babies born to lamivudine-treated mothers developed anti-HBs compared with only 61% of babies who received HBIG and vaccine at birth. Although HBV is present in breast milk, several studies have demonstrated that the risk of HBV transmission is not increased by breast feeding regardless of the E-antigen status or the level of serum HBV DNA in the mother.[84–86]

REFERENCES

1. Alter MJ. Epidemiology and prevention of hepatitis B. Semin Liver Dis 2003;23: 39–46.

2. Lavanchy D. Hepatitis B virus epidemiology, disease burden, treatment, and current and emerging prevention and control measures. J Viral Hepat 2004;11: 97–107.
3. Chu CJ, Keeffe EB, Han SH, et al. Hepatitis B virus genotypes in the United States: results of a nationwide study. Gastroenterology 2003;125:444–51.
4. Schreiber GB, Busch MP, Kleinman SH, et al. The risk of transfusion-transmitted viral infections. The Retrovirus Epidemiology Donor Study. N Engl J Med 1996; 334:1685–90.
5. Mast EE, Weinbaum CM, Fiore AE, et al. A comprehensive immunization strategy to eliminate transmission of hepatitis B virus infection in the United States. MMWR Recomm Rep 2006;55:RR-16.
6. Jiles RB, Daniels D, Yusuf HR, et al. Undervaccination with hepatitis B vaccine: missed opportunities or choice? Am J Prev Med 2001;20(Suppl 4):75–83.
7. Ferrante JM, Winston DG, Chen PH, et al. Family physicians' knowledge and screening of chronic hepatitis and liver cancer. Fam Med 2008;40:345–51.
8. Scott RM, Snitbhan R, Bancroft WH, et al. Experimental transmission of hepatitis B virus by semen and saliva. J Infect Dis 1980;142:67–71.
9. Alter HJ, Seeff LB, Kaplan PM, et al. Type B hepatitis: the infectivity of blood positive for e antigen and DNA polymerase after accidental needlestick exposure. N Engl J Med 1976;295:909–13.
10. Bond WW, Favero MS, Petersen NJ, et al. Survival of hepatitis B virus after drying and storage for one week. Lancet 1981;1(8219):550–1.
11. Goldstein ST, Alter MJ, Williams IT, et al. Incidence and risk factors for acute hepatitis B in the United States, 1982–1998: implications for vaccination programs. J Infect Dis 2002;185:713–9.
12. Koff RS, Slavin MM, Connelly JD, et al. Contagiousness of acute hepatitis B. Secondary attack rates in household contacts. Gastroenterology 1977;72: 297–300.
13. Bernier RH, Sampliner R, Gerety R, et al. Hepatitis B infection in households of chronic carriers of hepatitis B surface antigen: factors associated with prevalence of infection. Am J Epidemiol 1982;116:199–211.
14. MacKellar DA, Valleroy LA, Secura GM, et al. Young Men's Survey Study Group. Two decades after vaccine license: hepatitis B immunization and infection among young men who have sex with men. Am J Public Health 2001;91:965–71.
15. Levine OS, Vlahov D, Brookmeyer R, et al. Differences in the incidence of hepatitis B and human immunodeficiency virus infections among injecting drug users. J Infect Dis 1996;173:579–83.
16. Steinberg SC, Alter HJ, Leventhal BG. The risk of hepatitis transmission to family contacts of leukemia patients. J Pediatr 1975;87:753–6.
17. Perrillo RP, Strang S, Lowry OH. Different operating conditions affect risk of hepatitis B virus infection at two residential institutions for the mentally disabled. Am J Epidemiol 1986;123:690–8.
18. Steffen R. Risks of hepatitis B for travellers. Vaccine 1990;8(Suppl):S31–2.
19. Alter MJ, Favero MS, Maynard JE. Impact of infection control strategies on the incidence of dialysis-associated hepatitis in the United States. J Infect Dis 1986;153:1149–51.
20. Woodruff BA, Moyer LA, O'Rourke KM, et al. Blood exposure and the risk of hepatitis B virus infection in firefighters. J Occup Med 1993;35:1048–54.
21. Mahoney FJ, Stewart K, Hu H, et al. Progress toward the elimination of hepatitis B virus transmission among health care workers in the United States. Arch Intern Med 1997;157:2601–5.

22. Treichel U, Meyer zum Büschenfelde KH, Stockert RJ, et al. The asialoglycoprotein receptor mediates hepatic binding and uptake of natural hepatitis B virus particles derived from viraemic carriers. J Gen Virol 1994;75:3021–9.
23. Glebe D, Urban S. Viral and cellular determinants involved in hepadnaviral entry. World J Gastroenterol 2007;13:22–38.
24. Barker LF, Murray R. Relationship of virus dose to incubation time of clinical hepatitis and time of appearance of hepatitis-associated antigen. Am J Med Sci 1972; 263(1):27–33.
25. Krugman S, Overby LR, Mushahwar IK, et al. Viral hepatitis type B. Studies on natural history and prevention re-examined. N Engl J Med 1979;300:101–6.
26. Hoofnagle JH, DiBisceglie AM. Serologic diagnosis of acute and chronic viral hepatitis. Semin Liver Dis 1991;11:73–83.
27. McMahon BJ, Alward WL, Hall DB, et al. Acute hepatitis B virus infection: relation of age to the clinical expression of disease and subsequent development of the carrier state. J Infect Dis 1985;151:599–603.
28. Biswas R, Tabor E, Hsia CC, et al. Comparative sensitivity of HBV NATs and HBsAg assays for detection of acute HBV infection. Transfusion 2003;43:788–98.
29. Jackson BR, Busch MP, Stramer SL, et al. The cost-effectiveness of NAT for HIV, HCV, and HBV in whole-blood donations. Transfusion 2003;43:721–9.
30. Perrillo RP, Chau KH, Overby LR, et al. Anti-hepatitis B core immunoglobulin M in the serologic evaluation of hepatitis B virus infection and simultaneous infection with type B, delta agent, and non-A, non-B viruses. Gastroenterology 1983;85: 163–7.
31. Carman WF, Jacyna MR, Hadziyannis S, et al. Mutation preventing formation of hepatitis B e antigen in patients with chronic hepatitis B infection. Lancet 1989; 2(8663):588–91.
32. Funk ML, Rosenberg DM, Lok AS. World-wide epidemiology of HBeAg-negative chronic hepatitis B and associated precore and core promoter variants. J Viral Hepat 2002;9:52–61.
33. Huang CF, Lin SS, Ho YC, et al. The immune response induced by hepatitis B virus principal antigens. Cell Mol Immunol 2006;3:97–106.
34. Chu CJ, Keeffe EB, Han SH, et al. US HBV Epidemiology Study Group. Prevalence of HBV precore/core promoter variants in the United States. Hepatology 2003;38:619–28.
35. Gish RG, Locarnini S. Genotyping and genetic sequencing in clinical practice. Clin Liver Dis 2007;11:761–95.
36. Rehermann B. Immune responses in hepatitis B virus infection. Semin Liver Dis 2003;23:21–37.
37. Tur-Kaspa R, Teicher L, Laub O, et al. Alpha interferon suppresses hepatitis B virus enhancer activity and reduces viral gene transcription. J Virol 1990;64:1821–4.
38. Rehermann B, Fowler P, Sidney J, et al. The cytotoxic T lymphocyte response to multiple hepatitis B virus polymerase epitopes during and after acute viral hepatitis. J Exp Med 1995;181:1047–58.
39. Webster GJ, Reignat S, Maini MK, et al. Incubation phase of acute hepatitis B in man: dynamic of cellular immune mechanisms. Hepatology 2000;32:1117–24.
40. Maini MK, Boni C, Ogg GS, et al. Direct ex vivo analysis of hepatitis B virus-specific CD8(+) T cells associated with the control of infection. Gastroenterology 1999;117:1386–96.
41. Diepolder HM, Jung MC, Wierenga E, et al. Anergic TH1 clones specific for hepatitis B virus (HBV) core peptides are inhibitory to other HBV core-specific CD4+ T cells in vitro. J Virol 1996;70:7540–8.

42. Penna A, Artini M, Cavalli A, et al. Long-lasting memory T cell responses following self-limited acute hepatitis B. J Clin Invest 1996;98:1185–94.

43. Rehermann B, Lau D, Hoofnagle JH, et al. Cytotoxic T lymphocyte responsiveness after resolution of chronic hepatitis B virus infection. J Clin Invest 1996;97: 1655–65.

44. Michalak TI, Pasquinelli C, Guilhot S, et al. Hepatitis B virus persistence after recovery from acute viral hepatitis. J Clin Invest 1994;94:907.

45. Hyams KC. Risks of chronicity following acute hepatitis B virus infection: a review. Clin Infect Dis 1995;20:992–1000.

46. Lee WM. Etiologies of acute liver failure. Semin Liver Dis 2008;28:142–50.

47. Shukla NB, Poles MA. Hepatitis B virus infection: co-infection with hepatitis C virus, hepatitis D virus, and human immunodeficiency virus. Clin Liver Dis 2004;8:445–60.

48. Wai CT, Fontana RJ, Polson J, et al. US Acute Liver Failure Study Group. Clinical outcome and virological characteristics of hepatitis B-related acute liver failure in the United States. J Viral Hepat 2005;12:192–8.

49. Sagnelli E, Coppola N, Pisaturo M, et al. HBV superinfection in HCV chronic carriers: a disease that is frequently severe but associated with the eradication of HCV. Hepatology 2009;49:1090–7.

50. Caredda F, Rossi E, d'Arminio Monforte A, et al. Hepatitis B virus-associated co-infection and superinfection with delta agent: indistinguishable disease with different outcome. J Infect Dis 1985;151:925–8.

51. Hoofnagle JH, Dusheiko GM, Seeff LB, et al. Seroconversion from hepatitis B e antigen to antibody in chronic type B hepatitis. Ann Intern Med 1981;94: 744–8.

52. Liaw YF, Chu CM, Su IJ, et al. Clinical and histological events preceding hepatitis B e antigen seroconversion in chronic type B hepatitis. Gastroenterology 1983; 84:216–9.

53. Hsu YS, Chien RN, Yeh CT, et al. Long-term outcome after spontaneous HBeAg seroconversion in patients with chronic hepatitis B. Hepatology 2002; 35:1522–7.

54. Fattovich G, Rugge M, Brollo L, et al. Clinical, virologic and histologic outcome following seroconversion from HBeAg to anti-HBe in chronic hepatitis type B. Hepatology 1986;6:167–72.

55. Nair S, Perrillo RP. Serum alanine aminotransferase flares during interferon treatment of chronic hepatitis B: is sustained clearance of HBV DNA dependent on levels of pretreatment viremia? Hepatology 2001;34:1021–6.

56. Perrillo RP. Current treatment of chronic hepatitis B: benefits and limitations. Semin Liver Dis 2005;25(Suppl 1):20–8.

57. Lok AS, Liang RH, Chiu EK, et al. Reactivation of hepatitis B virus replication in patients receiving cytotoxic therapy. Report of a prospective study. Gastroenterology 1991;100:182–8.

58. Loomba R, Rowley A, Wesley R, et al. Systematic review: the effect of preventive lamivudine on hepatitis B reactivation during chemotherapy. Ann Intern Med 2008;148:519–28.

59. Laskus T, Slusarczyk J, Cianciara J, et al. Exacerbation of chronic active hepatitis type B after short-term corticosteroid therapy resulting in fatal liver failure. Am J Gastroenterol 1990;85:1414–7.

60. Lubel JS, Testro AG, Angus PW. Hepatitis B virus reactivation following immuno-suppressive therapy: guidelines for prevention and management. Intern Med J 2007;37:705–12.

61. Esteve M, Saro C, González-Huix F, et al. Chronic hepatitis B reactivation following infliximab therapy in Crohn's disease patients: need for primary prophylaxis. Gut 2004;53:1363–5.

62. Ito S, Nakazono K, Murasawa A, et al. Development of fulminant hepatitis B (precore variant mutant type) after the discontinuation of low-dose methotrexate therapy in a rheumatoid arthritis patient. Arthritis Rheum 2001;44:339–42.

63. Lee WC, Wu MJ, Cheng CH, et al. Lamivudine is effective for the treatment of reactivation of hepatitis B virus and fulminant hepatic failure in renal transplant recipients. Am J Kidney Dis 2001;38:1074–81.

64. Rizzetto M. Hepatitis D: thirty years after. J Hepatol 2009;50:1043–50.

65. Wu JC, Chen TZ, Huang YS, et al. Natural history of hepatitis D viral superinfection: significance of viremia detected by polymerase chain reaction. Gastroenterology 1995;108:796–802.

66. André FE. Summary of safety and efficacy data on a yeast-derived hepatitis B vaccine. Am J Med 1989;87(Suppl 3A):14S–20S.

67. Zajac BA, West DJ, McAleer WJ, et al. Overview of clinical studies with hepatitis B vaccine made by recombinant DNA. J Infect 1986;13(Suppl A):39–45.

68. Hsu HY, Chang MH, Chen DS, et al. Baseline seroepidemiology of hepatitis B virus infection in children in Taipei, 1984: a study just before mass hepatitis B vaccination program in Taiwan. J Med Virol 1986;18:301–7.

69. Ni YH, Chang MH, Huang LM, et al. Hepatitis B virus infection in children and adolescents in a hyperendemic area: 15 years after mass hepatitis B vaccination. Ann Intern Med 2001;135:796–800.

70. Kramer ES, Hofmann C, Smith PG, et al. Response to hepatitis A and B vaccine alone or in combination in patients with chronic hepatitis C virus and advanced fibrosis. Dig Dis Sci 2009;54:2016–25.

71. Wiedmann M, Liebert UG, Oesen U, et al. Decreased immunogenicity of recombinant hepatitis B vaccine in chronic hepatitis C. Hepatology 2000;31:230–4.

72. Fabrizi F, Dixit V, Magnini M, et al. Meta-analysis: intradermal vs. intramuscular vaccination against hepatitis B virus in patients with chronic kidney disease. Aliment Pharmacol Ther 2006;24:497–506.

73. Landrum ML, Huppler Hullsiek K, Ganesan A, et al. Hepatitis B vaccine responses in a large U.S. military cohort of HIV-infected individuals: another benefit of HAART in those with preserved CD4 count. Vaccine 2009;27:4731–8.

74. Yuen MF, Lim WL, Cheng CC, et al. Twelve-year follow-up of a prospective randomized trial of hepatitis B recombinant DNA yeast vaccine versus plasma-derived vaccine without booster doses in children. Hepatology 1999;29:924–7.

75. Lu CY, Chiang BL, Chi WK, et al. Waning immunity to plasma-derived hepatitis B vaccine and the need for boosters 15 years after neonatal vaccination. Hepatology 2004;40:1415–20.

76. Francis DP, Hadler SC, Thompson SE, et al. The prevention of hepatitis B with vaccine. Report of the centers for disease control multi-center efficacy trial among homosexual men. Ann Intern Med 1982;97:362–6.

77. Szmuness W, Stevens CE, Harley EJ, et al. Hepatitis B vaccine: demonstration of efficacy in a controlled clinical trial in a high-risk population in the United States. N Engl J Med 1980;303:833–41.

78. Quinnan GV Jr, Wells MA, Wittek AE, et al. Inactivation of human T-cell lymphotropic virus, type III by heat, chemicals, and irradiation. Transfusion 1986;26:481–3.

79. Miyake Y, Iwasaki Y, Takaki A, et al. Lamivudine treatment improves the prognosis of fulminant hepatitis B. Intern Med 2008;47:1293–9.
80. Tillmann HL, Hadem J, Leifeld L, et al. Safety and efficacy of lamivudine in patients with severe acute or fulminant hepatitis B, a multicenter experience. J Viral Hepat 2006;13:256–63.
81. Xu DZ, Yan YP, Choi BC, et al. Risk factors and mechanism of transplacental transmission of hepatitis B virus: a case-control study. J Med Virol 2002;67:20–6.
82. Burk RD, Hwang LY, Ho GY, et al. Outcome of perinatal hepatitis B virus exposure is dependent on maternal virus load. J Infect Dis 1994;170:1418–23.
83. Xu WM, Cui YT, Wang L. Efficacy and safety of lamivudine in late pregnancy for the prevention of mother-child transmission of hepatitis B: a multicenter, random-ized, placebo double-blind, placebo controlled study. Hepatology 2004;40:272A.
84. Beasley RP, Stevens CE, Shiao IS, et al. Evidence against breast-feeding as a mechanism for vertical transmission of hepatitis B. Lancet 1975;2(7938):740–1.
85. de Martino M, Appendino C, Resti M, et al. Should hepatitis B surface antigen positive mothers breast feed? Arch Dis Child 1985;60:972–4.
86. Hill JB, Sheffield JS, Kim MJ, et al. Risk of hepatitis B transmission in breast-fed infants of chronic hepatitis B carriers. Obstet Gynecol 2002;99:1049–52.

Health Care–Associated Transmission of Hepatitis B & C Viruses in Dental Care (Dentistry)

Fariba S. Younai, DDS

KEYWORDS

- Dentistry • Transmission • Hepatitis B
- Hepatitis C • Prevention

Of the nine million health care providers practicing in the United States, 608,000 are dental health care personnel (DHCP), including 176,000 dentists, 217,000 dental hygienists, and 362,00 dental assistants.[1] It is projected that by 2016, this number will grow to approximately 755,000 DHCP. Dental patients and DHCP are at risk for infection with microorganisms that either colonize or infect the oral cavity and the respiratory tract or may be present in the oral tissues from the circulating blood.[2] Among these, there are several blood-borne viral diseases, including infections caused by hepatitis B virus (HBV) and hepatitis C virus (HCV).[3] Dentistry is considered as one of the health professions with the highest risk of HBV exposure, with infection rates among dentists that are 3 to 10 times higher than the general population.[4–9] Historically and prior to the institution of mandatory HBV vaccination for health care workers, the prevalence rate for HBV markers among dentists was shown to be 16% to 28%, [10,11] and several clusters of HBV transmission from infected dentists and oral surgeons to patients were reported.[12–21] In terms of hepatitis C, one longitudinal cohort study showed a slightly higher prevalence rate for carrier state among DHCP compared to the other health care workers in the study (1.7% vs 1.4%).[11] In dental care settings, microorganisms can be transmitted through direct contact with contaminated instruments or surfaces, splash or spray of infectious fluids or materials in the mucosa of the eyes or mouth, and by inhalation of airborne infectious agents.[2,22]

HEPATITIS B EPIDEMIOLOGY

An estimated 400 million people have chronic HBV infection worldwide.[13] Every year, an estimated 900,000 people die of acute hepatitis, liver cirrhosis, or hepatocellular

Division of Oral Biology and Medicine, Department of Oral Medicine & Orofacial Pain, UCLA School of Dentistry, 10833 Le Conte Avenue, Los Angeles, CA 90095-1668, USA
E-mail address: fyounai@dentistry.ucla.edu

Clin Liver Dis 14 (2010) 93–104
doi:10.1016/j.cld.2009.11.010
1089-3261/10/$ – see front matter © 2010 Elsevier Inc. All rights reserved.

carcinoma caused by chronic HBV infection.[23] In the United States, it is estimated that between 800,000 to 1.4 million people have chronic HBV infection, and each year an estimated 50,000 new infections occur.[24] Community HBV transmission involves exposure to infectious body fluids such as blood, semen, and saliva, mostly through vertical, sexual, and parenteral modes. The current HBV incidence rate in the United States reflects a significant drop compared to mid-1980s, primarily because of aggressive vaccination of infants and high-risk populations.[24] Currently, heterosexual transmission accounts for approximately 39% of new HBV infections among adults; transmission among men who have sex with men comprises approximately 24% of cases, and injection drug use (IDU) accounts for approximately 16% of new HBV infections.[25] Other adult cases of chronic HBV infection are seen among household contacts of other chronically infected individuals, patients on hemodialysis, travelers to areas with high endemic rates for hepatitis B, and occupational exposures.[25] In health care settings, needle sticks or other sharps injuries are responsible for most occupational HBV transmissions. In addition, HBV has been shown to be able to survive for as much as 1 week on environmental surfaces.[26] Therefore, lapses in infection control practices and poor barrier techniques account for the remainder of transmission cases among health care workers and also may be responsible for many cases of nosocomial or patient-to-patient transmissions.[27–29]

CLINICAL FEATURES AND NATURAL HISTORY OF HBV INFECTION

HBV, a DNA virus from the *Hepadnaviridae* family, is capable of causing hepatic inflammation and the clinical syndrome of acute jaundice.[30] After an exposure event involving a susceptible host, the virus reaches the liver through the bloodstream and successfully establishes an infection in hepatocytes. HBV infection occurs with an average incubation period of 90 days (range: 60 to 150 days) from exposure to the onset of jaundice and 60 days (range: 40 to 90 days) from exposure to the onset of abnormal serum alanine aminotransferase (ALT) levels.[31,32] Newly acquired HBV infection may be symptomatic. For instance, in infants, children aged younger than 5 years, and immunosuppressed adults, acute infection is typically asymptomatic, whereas 30% to 50% of children aged *over* 5 years and adults have initial clinical signs or symptoms.[33] These may include signs of hepatic disease such as clinical jaundice, anorexia, malaise, nausea, vomiting, abdominal pain, and extrahepatic signs like skin rashes, arthralgias, and arthritis.[30] A small proportion of patients may develop severe acute hepatitis B. The risk for severe acute hepatitis B may be increased in persons who are coinfected with hepatitis C or D.[33] The fatality rate among persons with reported cases of acute hepatitis B is 0.5% to 1.0%, with the highest rates in adults aged over 60 years.[25]

The earliest marker of infection, appearing within 4 to 10 weeks after the exposure, is hepatitis B surface antigen (HBsAg), a glycoprotein associated with the surface of the viral envelope.[23] The hepatitis B virion contains two other major antigens in its core, along with a partially double-stranded DNA and a DNA polymerase enzyme. One of the core antigens, hepatitis B core antigen (HBcAg), is not readily detectable in blood. The other, hepatitis B e antigen (HBeAg) appears in blood shortly after the HBsAg and is associated with significant liver inflammation manifested by a marked increase in serum transaminases and bilirubin.[34] The presence of HBeAg generally indicates high levels of HBV DNA in the blood.[25]

The first humoral response to HBV infection is the development of immunoglobulin (Ig) M antibody to HBcAg (anti-HBc), which is detectable in blood shortly after the appearance of HBsAg. Shortly thereafter, this antibody is replaced with IgG anti-HBc, remaining in blood for years after the infection. The next events in individuals who clear the infection involves development of anti-HBe, marking the end of active liver disease and ultimately anti-HBs, indicating recovery and immunity.[34] Approximately 95% of primary infections in adults with normal immune status follow a self-limited course and involve the elimination of the HBV from blood and subsequent lasting immunity to reinfection (development of anti-HBs).[23] A small proportion of individuals who clear the infection will have intermittent low levels of HBV DNA in serum referred to as latent hepatitis B. In these infected persons, progression to liver disease is unlikely, but viral reactivation may occur with severe immunosuppression.[23]

Chronic infection occurs in about 5% of infected individuals over the age 5, in approximately 30% of infected children aged less than 5 years, and in almost all infected infants, with continuing viral replication in the liver and persistent viremia.[25,33] Primary infections become chronic more frequently in immunosuppressed persons (eg, hemodialysis patients and persons with human immunodeficiency virus [HIV] infection) [25,35,36] and persons with diabetes.[25,37] Persons who were infected as adults or adolescents and have developed chronic HBV infection eventually enter the inactive carrier phase, whereas in those infected at birth or in early childhood, the disease continues to progress. The inactive carrier state is associated with clearing the HBeAg and developing anti-HBe (HBeAg seroconversion) with undetectable or low levels of HBV DNA, normalization of serum ALT levels, and reduced liver inflammation.[23] It is noteworthy that HBV DNA remains present in the blood during the inactive carrier phase, but at lower levels than during the active phase.[23]

Overall, approximately 25% of persons who become chronically infected during childhood and 15% of those who become chronically infected after childhood die prematurely from cirrhosis or liver cancer; most remain asymptomatic until the onset of cirrhosis or end-stage liver disease.[25,38] In chronically HBV-infected individuals, medical evaluation and regular monitoring are critical to ensuring sustained suppression of HBV replication and remission of liver disease. Currently, the therapeutic agents approved by the US Food and Drug Administration (FDA) for treating chronic hepatitis B include interferons (interferon-α2b and peginterferon-α2a) and nucleoside or nucleotide analogues (lamivudine, adefovir, entecavir, tenofovir, and telbivudine).[13] The major goals of anti-HBV therapy are to prevent progressive liver disease, cirrhosis, liver failure, and subsequent development of hepatocellular carcinoma and death. It is not yet clear if the short-term positive results reported by anti-HBV therapies will, in the long term, provide protection against liver failure and carcinoma development. Periodic screening with ultrasonography and alfa-fetoprotein has been demonstrated to enhance early detection of hepatocellular carcinoma.[39]

HEPATITIS B AND THE DENTAL CARE SETTING

In dental care settings, microorganisms can be transmitted through

  Direct contact with blood, oral fluids, or other patient materials
  Indirect contact with contaminated objects (eg, instruments, equipment, or environmental surfaces)
  Contact of conjunctival, nasal, or oral mucosa with droplets (eg, spatter) containing microorganisms generated from an infected person and propelled a short distance (eg, by coughing, sneezing, or talking)

Inhalation of airborne microorganisms that can remain suspended in the air for long periods.[22]

For many of these exposures, transmission of HBV is very plausible because of contamination with blood and saliva. It has been shown that both infectious viruses and HBsAg particles are present in saliva; however, the number of infectious viruses is very low even in HBsAg-positive blood.[40] Generally, percutaneous injuries with sharp instruments such as cutting instruments and anesthetic needles are the most common source of occupational exposures in dentistry.[10,41–45] A survey of dental practitioners by the American Dental Association showed that private practitioners experience an average of 3.2 injuries per year.[44] This rate has been reported to be much higher for dental education institutions[46] and with an approximate 0.3% to 0.5% of the US population being chronically infected with hepatitis B, the great potential for transmission of HBV to the DHCP is quite evident. In fact, some of the earlier prevalence studies showed the prevalence of HBV serologic markers among dentists to range from 16% to 28%.[10,11] Since the early 1980s, the transmission of HBV to DHCP has declined dramatically (prevalence of serologic markers dropped to 9% in 1992), mostly as a result of better compliance with HBV vaccination and improved infection control practices.[47]

Several reports, published between 1970 to 1987, described nine clusters of HBV transmission from three infected general dentists and six oral surgeons to their patients.[12–21] The number of patients varied in each cluster and was as high as 55[16] and 37,[14] both involving oral surgeons, to 3[19] and 4,[21] from an oral surgeon and a general practitioner. No such transmission has been reported since 1987 in dentistry, most likely because of more widespread HBV vaccination of DHCP, universal glove use, and implementation of the 1991 Occupational Safety and Health Administration (OSHA) Bloodborne Pathogens Standard.[48] One case of patient-to-patient transmission has been documented where the exact mechanism of transmission was unproven.[49]

HEPATITIS C EPIDEMIOLOGY

HCV, first identified in 1989,[50] is now considered responsible for chronic infection in 3% of the world population, approximately 170 million individuals.[50,51] Globally 3 to 4 million new infections occur every year.[51] In the United States, an estimated 3.2 million people are living with chronic HCV infection, with roughly 19,000 new infections reported in 2006 alone.[24] The most efficient mode of HCV transmission is through blood exposure. Therefore, most cases (60%) of infections in the United States are seen among injection drug users. Of persons injecting drugs for at least 5 years, 60% to 80% are infected with HCV, compared with about 30% infected with HIV.[52] Donor deferrals and screening of blood and blood products for HCV antibodies and surrogate markers (ALT), which began in 1990, have been effective in significantly reducing the number of new cases of post-transfusion infections.[53] As of 2001, the risk of HCV infection from a unit of transfused blood is less than one per million transfused units.[52] Sexual transmission is responsible for 15% of the reported cases in the United States.[52] A total of 5% of exposures are caused by hemodialysis, employment in the health care field, and birth to an HCV-infected mother; for 10% of cases, no recognized source for infection has been identified.[52] It has been shown that HCV in plasma can survive drying and environmental exposure to room temperature for at least 16 hours,[54] suggesting a potential for transmission through blood contamination of environmental surfaces and inanimate objects.

CLINICAL FEATURES AND NATURAL HISTORY OF HCV INFECTION

HCV, an RNA virus of the *Flaviviridae* family, has 6 genotypes and more than 50 subtypes.[55] Genotype 1 accounts for 70% to 75% of all HCV infections in the United States and is associated with a lower rate of response to treatment.[56,57] HCV replicates preferentially in hepatocytes but is not directly cytopathic, leading to persistent infection.[55]

The incubation period for acute HCV infection is 1 to 3 weeks. Within an average of 4 to 12 weeks, HCV RNA can be detected in blood and corresponds to the onset of symptoms and elevated serum ALT levels. Acute infection can be severe but rarely is fulminant.[55] Symptoms are uncommon but can include malaise, weakness, anorexia, and jaundice.[24] Symptoms usually subside after several weeks as ALT levels decline. An average of 60% to 70% of infections lead to a chronic carrier state; 10% to 20% of chronic carriers develop liver cirrhosis, and 1% to 5% develop hepatocellular carcinoma.[58] Older age at time of infection, male gender, diabetes, alcohol use, and co-infection with HIV or HBV appear to increase the risk of progressive liver disease.[23,52,55,59] Patients with chronic hepatitis C can present with extrahepatic manifestations such as rheumatoid arthritis, keratoconjunctivitis sicca, lichen planus, glomerulonephritis, lymphoma, and essential mixed cryoglobulinemia.[55] HCV-associated chronic liver disease is the most frequent indication for liver transplantation among adults.[52]

During chronic infection, HCV RNA reaches high levels, generally ranging from 10^5 to 10^7 IU/mL. Ultrasensitive enzyme immunoassays (EIAs) that can detect HCV antibodies are used for screening at-risk populations and are recommended as the initial test for patients with clinical liver disease. A negative EIA test rules out chronic HCV infection in immune-competent patients, but patients on hemodialysis and patients with immune deficiencies may have false-negative EIAs.[55] For these patients, an assay for HCV RNA (target amplification, polymerase chain reaction [PCR], or signal amplification techniques like branched DNA) is necessary for diagnosis of chronic infection.

The goal of HVC treatment is to prevent complications of chronic infection. This is principally achieved by eradication of infection. Current treatment standards involve the use of pegylated interferon (alfa-2a and alfa-2b) in combination with ribavirin.[60–62] HCV genotype 1 requires a longer course of treatment with pegylated interferon and higher dose of ribavirin than other genotypes.[60] Early viral response demonstrated by a rapid drop in the HCV viral load is predictive of sustained viral response (at 6 months).[60] Treatment is recommended for patients with an increased risk of developing cirrhosis. These patients include those with detectable HCV RNA levels (higher than 50 IU/mL), a liver biopsy indicative of portal or bridging fibrosis, or moderate inflammation and necrosis. Most also have persistently elevated ALT values.[60,61]

HEPATITIS C AND DENTAL CARE SETTING

Approximately, 50% of HCV-infected individuals have HCV-RNA in their saliva.[63] In addition, there is a direct relationship between the presence of HCV in saliva and the plasma HCV load.[63–65] Studies also have shown HCV particles to be present in oral epithelial cells.[66,67] These findings may suggest that HCV would be transmissible through household contacts, explaining the roughly 10% of new cases where no specific mode of transmission can be identified.[52] It also may imply that the dental environment may be at especially high risk for occupational HCV transmission. Evidence, however, suggests that the infectivity of HCV in saliva may be very low. As reviewed by Ferreiro and colleagues,[68] studies have not been able to demonstrate a high capacity for infectivity by HCV particles found in different oral compartments.

Also, there is no epidemiologic evidence for HCV transmission through orogenital exposure, kissing, or household contact. Moreover, the prevalence rates of DHCP have been shown to be only slightly higher than the general population.[11] One study of general dentists and oral surgeons showed anti-HCV antibodies in 2% of oral surgeons and 0.7% of general practitioners.[69] To date, no case of transmission from an HCV-infected dentist to his or her patients has been reported.[70]

OCCUPATIONAL EXPOSURES TO HBV AND HCV IN DENTISTRY

In June 2001, the Centers for Disease Control and Prevention (CDC) published its last up-dated recommendation for the management of occupational HIV, HBV, and HCV exposures, and recommendations for postexposure prophylaxis.[40] Since then, other updates have been published to include new antiretroviral drugs for postexposure prophylaxis against HIV, but the recommendations for HBV and HCV have remained the same.[71] This section provides a summary of the US Public Health Service (PHS) guidelines and also includes specific recommendations for infection control in dental settings.[72]

HBV infection is a well recognized occupational risk for DHCP.[4–9] For each exposure incident involving an HBV-infected source patient, the risk of HBV infection is related directly to the degree of contact with blood or other infected body fluids and the HBeAg status of the source person.[72] The risk of developing clinical hepatitis after exposure to blood that is both HBsAg- and HBeAg-positive has been shown to range from 22% to 31%; the risk of developing serologic evidence of HBV infection is 37% to 62%. In contrast, the risk of developing clinical hepatitis from a needle contaminated with HBsAg-positive, HBeAg-negative blood is about 1% to 6%, and the risk of developing serologic evidence of HBV infection is 23% to 37%.[73] Recent data indicate fluctuating levels of HBV DNA among hepatitis B carriers.[74] Therefore an assessment of the viral DNA load, regardless of the HBeAg status, may be necessary to assess a person's degree of infectivity.[75]

Percutaneous injuries with sharp dental instruments and hollow bore anesthetic needles are among the most efficient modes of HBV transmission. However, direct or indirect blood or body fluid exposures that can inoculate HBV into cutaneous scratches, abrasions, burns, other lesions, or on mucosal surfaces have been documented.[27–29] This type of exposure may not only be immediate, as HBV has been demonstrated to survive in dried blood at room temperature on environmental surfaces for at least 1 week.[26] The potential for HBV transmission through contact with environmental surfaces has been demonstrated in investigations of HBV outbreaks among patients and staff of hemodialysis units.[76–78]

HCV is not transmitted efficiently through occupational exposures to blood. The average incidence of anti-HCV seroconversion after accidental percutaneous exposure from an HCV-positive source is 1.8% (range: 0% to 7%).[79–82] Transmission rarely occurs from mucous membrane exposures to blood, and no transmission has been documented from intact or nonintact skin exposures to blood.[83,84] Although it has been shown that HCV can survive on environmental surfaces for a few hours,[54] epidemiologic data do not support a significant risk for HCV transmission in the health care setting through environmental contamination with blood.[43,85] The risk for transmission from exposure to fluids or tissues other than HCV-infected blood also has not been quantified but is expected to be low.

POSTEXPOSURE PROPHYLAXIS

For percutaneous or mucosal exposures to blood, factors to be considered are the HBsAg status of the source and the hepatitis B vaccination and vaccine-response status of the exposed person. Such exposures usually involve persons for whom hepatitis B vaccination is recommended. Any blood or body fluid exposure to an unvaccinated person should lead to initiation of the hepatitis B vaccine series.

If a DHCP has not been vaccinated against HBV, or if he or she has started the vaccination series but has not completed it, or is known not to have responded to the initial vaccination series, then a single dose of hepatitis B immunoglobulin (HBIG) should be administered as soon as possible after exposure (preferably within 24 hours). The effectiveness of HBIG when administered more than 7 days after exposure is unknown. For all these individuals hepatitis B vaccine is indicated:

To initiate the series for the nonvaccinated
To complete the series for those who have already received one or two doses
To repeat the vaccination series for the nonresponders.

The vaccine also should be administered as soon as possible (preferably within 24 hours), and it can be administered simultaneously with HBIG at a separate site (vaccine always should be administered in the deltoid muscle).

DHCP exposed to an HCV-positive source should receive baseline testing for anti-HCV and ALT activity and also follow-up testing (eg, at 4 to 6 months) for anti-HCV and ALT activity (if earlier diagnosis of HCV infection is desired, testing for HCV RNA may be performed at 4 to 6 weeks). Confirm all anti-HCV results reported positive by EIA using supplemental anti-HCV testing by recombinant immunoblot assay (RIBA II; Ortho Diagnostics, Raritan, NJ, USA). The exposed DHCP should be counseled on the risk for HCV infection and appropriate medical follow-up. They should be advised to refrain from donating blood, plasma, organs, tissue, or semen. The exposed person does not need to modify sexual practices or refrain from becoming pregnant.

Immunoglobulin and antiviral agents are not recommended for postexposure prophylaxis after exposure to HCV-positive blood. In addition, no guidelines exist for administration of therapy during the acute phase of HCV infection. Limited data, however, indicate that antiviral therapy might be beneficial when started early in the course of HCV infection. When HCV infection is identified early, the person should be referred for medical management to a specialist knowledgeable in this area.

No modifications to an exposed person's patient care responsibilities are necessary to prevent transmission to patients based solely on exposure to HBV- or HCV-positive blood. If an exposed person becomes acutely infected with HBV, the person should be evaluated for his or her medical status. No recommendations exist regarding restricting the professional activities of HCP with HCV infection. As recommended for all health care providers, DHCP who are chronically infected with HBV or HCV should follow all recommended infection control practices, including standard precautions and appropriate use of hand washing, protective barriers, and care in the use and disposal of needles and other sharp instruments.[86]

SUMMARY

The dental environment is associated with significant risk for HBV transmission and to a lesser degree for HCV exposure and infection. DCHP are required to receive hepatitis B vaccination and must follow infection control strategies that are consistent with standard precautions to reduce the risk for HCV transmission. For occupational exposures in dentistry, the latest PHS guidelines are used to properly guide postexposure evaluation and management of DHCP.

REFERENCES

1. Bureau of Labor Statistics. United States Department of Labor 2009. Occupational outlook handbook, 2008–2009 edition. Available at: http://www.bls.gov/oco/ocos072.htm. Accessed April 20, 2009.
2. Kohn WG, Collins AS, Cleveland JL, et al. Guidelines for infection control in dental health care settings. Morb Mort Weekly Rep 2003;52(RR17):1–61.
3. Sepkowitz KA. Occupationally acquired infections in health care workers: part II. Ann Intern Med 1996;25(11):917–28.
4. Mosley JW, White E. Viral hepatitis as an occupational hazard of dentists. J Am Dent Assoc 1975;90:992–7.
5. Mosley JW, Edwards VM, Casey G, et al. Hepatitis B virus infection in dentists. N Engl J Med 1975;293(15):729–34.
6. Feldman RE, Schiff ER. Hepatitis in dental professionals. JAMA 1975;232:1228–30.
7. Smith JL, Maynard JE, Berquist KR, et al. From the Centers for Disease Control: comparative risk of hepatitis B among physicians and dentists. J Infect Dis 1976;133(6):705–6.
8. Hollinger FB, Grander JW, Nickel FR, et al. Hepatitis B prevalence within a dental student population. J Am Dent Assoc 1977;94:521–7.
9. Wei RB, Lyman DO, Jackson RJ, et al. A hepatitis serosurvey of New York dentists. NY State Dent J 1977;43:587–90.
10. Schiff ER, Medina MD, Kline SN, et al. Veterans administration cooperative study of hepatitis and dentistry. J Am Dent Assoc 1986;113(3):390–6.
11. Gerberding JL. Incidence and prevalence of human immunodeficiency virus, hepatitis B, hepatitis C and cytomegalovirus among healthcare personnel at risk for blood exposure. Final report from a longitudinal study. J Infect Dis 1994;170(6):1410–7.
12. Levin ML, Maddrey WC, Wands JR, et al. Hepatitis B transmission by dentists. JAMA 1974;228:1139–40.
13. Williams SV, Pattison CP, Berquist KR. Dental infections with hepatitis B. JAMA 1975;232:1231–3.
14. Goodwin D, Fannin SL, McCracken BB. An oral surgeon related hepatitis B outbreak. California Morbidity, Infectious Disease Section, Department of Health 1976;14:21–6.
15. Watkins BJ. Viral hepatitis B: a special problem in prevention. J Am Soc Prev Dent 1976;6:9–13.
16. Rimland D, Parkin WE, Miller JB, et al. Hepatitis B outbreak traced to an oral surgeon. N Engl J Med 1977;296:953–8.
17. Hadler SC, Sorley DL, Acree KH, et al. An outbreak of hepatitis B in a dental practice. Ann Intern Med 1981;95:133–8.
18. Reingold AL, Kane MA, Murphy BL, et al. Transmission of hepatitis B by an oral surgeon. J Infect Dis 1982;145:262–3.
19. Ahtone J, Goodman RA. Hepatitis B and dental personnel: transmission to patients and prevention issues. J Am Dent Assoc 1983;106:219–22.
20. Shaw FE Jr, Barrett CL, Hamm R, et al. Lethal outbreak of hepatitis B in a dental practice. JAMA 1986;255:3260–4.
21. Centers for Disease Control and Prevention. Outbreak of hepatitis B associated with an oral surgeon—New Hampshire. Morb Mort Week Rep 1987;36:132–3.
22. Bolyard EA, Tablan OC, Williams WW, et al. Hospital Infection Control Practices Advisory Committee. Guideline for infection control in health care personnel, 1998. Am J Infect Control 1998;26:289–354.

23. Sorrell MF, Belongia EA, Costa J, et al. National Institutes of Health consensus development conference statement: management of hepatitis B. Ann Intern Med 2009;150(2):104–10.

24. Centers or Disease Control and Prevention. Division of Viral Hepatitis. ABCs of hepatitis fact sheet. Available at: www.cdc.gov/hepatitis. Accessed April 20, 2009.

25. Mast EE, Weinbaum CM, Fiore AE, et al. A comprehensive immunization strategy to eliminate transmission of hepatitis B virus infection in the United States. Recommendations of the Advisory Committee on Immunization Practices (ACIP) part II: immunization of adults. Morb Mort Weekly Rep 2006;55(RR16): 1–25.

26. Bond WW, Favero MS, Petersen NJ, et al. Survival of hepatitis B virus after drying and storage for one week [letter]. Lancet 1981;1:550–1.

27. Francis DP, Favero MS, Maynard JE. Transmission of hepatitis B virus. Semin Liver Dis 1981;1:27–32.

28. Favero MS, Maynard JE, Petersen NJ, et al. Hepatitis B antigen on environmental surfaces [letter]. Lancet 1973;2:1455.

29. Lauer JL, VanDrunen NA, Washburn JW, et al. Transmission of hepatitis B virus in clinical laboratory areas. J Infect Dis 1979;140:513–6.

30. Lemon SM, Newbold JE. Viral hepatitis. In: Holmes KK, Mårdh P-A, Sparling PF, editors. Sexually transmitted diseases. 2nd edition. New York: McGraw-Hill; 1990. p. 449.

31. Krugman S, Overby LR, Mushahwar IK, et al. Viral hepatitis, type B. Studies on natural history and prevention re-examined. N Engl J Med 1979;300:101–6.

32. Hoofnagle JH, DiBisceglie AM. Serologic diagnosis of acute and chronic viral hepatitis. Semin Liver Dis 1991;11:73–83.

33. McMahon BJ, Alward WL, Hall DB, et al. Acute hepatitis B virus infection: relation of age to the clinical expression of disease and subsequent development of the carrier state. J Infect Dis 1985;151:599–603.

34. Younai FS. Postexposure protocol. Dent Clin North Am 1996;40(2):457–86.

35. Hyams KC. Risks of chronicity following acute hepatitis B virus infection: a review. Clin Infect Dis 1995;20:992–1000.

36. Hadler SC, Judson FN, O'Malley PM, et al. Outcome of hepatitis B virus infection in homosexual men and its relation to prior human immunodeficiency virus infection. J Infect Dis 1991;163:454–9.

37. Polish LB, Shapiro CN, Bauer F, et al. Nosocomial transmission of hepatitis B virus-associated with the use of a spring-loaded finger-stick device. N Engl J Med 1992;326:721–5.

38. Goldstein ST, Zhou F, Hadler SC, et al. A mathematical model to estimate hepatitis B disease burden and vaccination impact. Int J Epidemiol 2005;34:1329–39.

39. Bruix J, Sherman M. Practice guidelines committee. American Association for the Study of Liver Disease (AASLD). Management of hepatocellular carcinoma. Hepatology 2005;42:1208–36.

40. Centers for Disease Control and Prevention. Updated U.S. public health service guidelines for the management of occupational exposures to HBV, HCV, and HIV and recommendations for postexposure prophylaxis. Morb Mort Weekly Rep 2001;50:1–52.

41. Cottone JA, Dillars RL, Dove SB. Frequency of percutaneous injuries in dental care providers [abstract]. J Dent Educ 1992;56:34.

42. Gonzalez CD, Pruhs RJ, Sampson E. Clinical occupational bloodborne exposure in a dental school. J Dent Educ 1994;58:217–20.

43. Polish LB, Tong MJ, Co RL, et al. Risk factors for hepatitis C virus infection among healthcare personnel in a community hospital. Am J Infect Control 1993;21: 196–200.
44. Siew C, Chang SB, Gruninger SE, et al. Self-reported percutaneous injuries in dentists: implications for HBV and HIV transmission risks. J Am Dent Assoc 1992;123:36–44.
45. Younai FS, Murphy DC, Kotelchuck D. Occupational exposures to blood in a dental teaching environment: results of a ten-year surveillance study. J Dent Educ 2001;65:436–48.
46. Kotelchuck D, Murphy D, Younai F. Impact of underreporting on the management of occupational bloodborne exposures in a dental teaching environment. J Dent Educ 2004;68:614–22.
47. Cleveland JL, Siew C, Lockwood SA, et al. Hepatitis B vaccination and infection among US dentists, 1983–1992. J Am Dent Assoc 1996;127: 1385–90.
48. US Department of Labor. Occupational health and safety administration. 29 CFR part 1910.1030. Occupational exposure to bloodborne pathogens; final rule. Fed Regist 1991;56:64004–182.
49. Redd JT, Baumbach J, Kohn W, et al. Patient-to patient transmission of hepatitis B virus associated with oral surgery. J Infect Dis 2007;195:1311–4.
50. Choo QL, Kuo G, Weiner AJ, et al. Isolation of cDNA clone derived from a blood-borne non-A, non-B viral hepatitis genome. Science 1989;244:359–62.
51. World Health Organization. Hepatitis C. Available at: http://www.who.int/mediacentre/factsheets/fs164/en/index.html. Accessed April 20, 2009.
52. Division of Viral Hepatitis, National Center for Infectious Disease Control and Prevention. National Hepatitis Prevention Strategy. A comprehensive strategy for the prevention and control of hepatitis C virus infections and its consequences 2001. p. 1–21. Available at: http://www.cdc.gov/hepatitis/HCV/Strategy/NatHepCPrevStrategy.htm. Accessed April 20, 2009.
53. Donahue JG, Muñoz A, Ness PM, et al. The declining risk of post-transfusion hepatitis C virus infection. N Engl J Med 1992;325:369–73.
54. Kamili S, Krawczynski K, McCaustland K, et al. Infectivity of hepatitis C virus in plasma after drying and storing at room temperature. Infect Control Hosp Epidemiol 2007;28:519–24.
55. National Institutes of Health. NIH consensus and state-of-the-science statements. Management of Hepatitis C: 2002. 2002;9(3):1–52. Available at: http://consensus.nih.gov/2002/2002HepatitisC2002116html.htm. Accessed April 20, 2009.
56. Fried MW, Shiffman ML, Reddy KR, et al. Peginterferon alfa-2a plus ribavirin for chronic hepatitis C virus infection. N Engl J Med 2002;347:975–82.
57. Manns MP, McHutchison JG, Gordon SC, et al. Peginterferon alfa-2b plus ribavirin compared with interferon alfa-2b plus ribavirin for initial treatment of chronic hepatitis C: a randomized trial. Lancet 2001;358(9286):958–65.
58. Alter MJ. The detection, transmission, and outcome of hepatitis C virus infection. Infect Agents Dis 1993;2:155–66.
59. Hu SX, Kyulo NL, Xia VW, et al. Factors associated with hepatic fibrosis in patients with chronic hepatitis C: a retrospective study of a large cohort of US patients. J Clin Gastroenterol 2009;43:758–64.
60. National Institutes of Health. National Institutes of Health consensus development conference statement: management of hepatitis C: 2002. Hepatology 2002;36: S3–20.

61. Strader DB, Wright T, Thomas DL, et al. American Association for the Study of Liver Diseases. Diagnosis, management, and treatment of hepatitis C. Hepatology 2004;39:1147–71.
62. Farrell GC. New hepatitis C guidelines for the Asia-Pacific region: APASL consensus statements on the diagnosis, management and treatment of hepatitis C virus infection. J Gastroenterol Hepatol 2007;22:607–10.
63. Hermida M, Ferreiro MC, Barral S, et al. Detection of HCV RNA in saliva of patients with hepatitis C virus infection by using a highly sensitive test. J Virol Methods 2002;101:29–35.
64. Fabris P, Infantolino D, Biasin MR, et al. High prevalence of HCV-RNA in the saliva fraction of patients with chronic hepatitis C infection but no evidence of HCV transmission among sexual partners. Infection 1999;27:86–91.
65. Belec L, Legoff J, Si-Mohamed A, et al. Mucosal humoral immune response to hepatitis C virus E1/E2 surface glycoproteins and cervicovaginal fluids from chronically-infected patients. J Hepatol 2003;38:833–42.
66. Arrieta JJ, Rodriguez-Iñigo E, Casqueiro M, et al. Detection of hepatitis C virus replication by in situ hybridization in epithelial cells of anti-hepatitis C virus-positive patients with and without oral lichen planus. Hepatology 2000;32:97–103.
67. Carrozzo M, Quadri R, Latorre P, et al. Molecular evidence that hepatitis C virus replicates in the oral mucosa. J Hepatol 2002;37:364–9.
68. Ferreiro MC, Dios PD, Scully C. Transmission of hepatitis C virus by saliva? Oral Dis 2005;11:230–5.
69. Thomas DL, Gruninger SE, Siew C, et al. Occupational risk of hepatitis C infections among general dentists and oral surgeons in North America. Am J Med 1996;100:41–5.
70. Mason BW, Cartwright J, Sandham S, et al. A patient notification exercise following infection control failures in a dental surgery. Braz Dent J 2008;205:E8.
71. Centers for Disease Control and Prevention. Updated US Public health service guidelines for the management of occupational exposures to HIV and recommendations for post-exposure prophylaxis. Morb Mort Weekly Rep 2005;54:1–17.
72. CDC. Guidelines for infection control in dental health care settings-2003. Morb Mort Week Report 2003;52:1–68.
73. Werner BG, Grady GF. Accidental hepatitis B surface antigen-positive inoculations: use of e-antigen to estimate infectivity. Ann Intern Med 1982;97:367–9.
74. Tedder RS, Ijaz S, Gilbert N, et al. Evidence for a dynamic host-parasite relationship in e-negative hepatitis B carriers. J Med Virol 2002;68:505–12.
75. Heptonstall J, Barnes J, Burton E, et al. Transmission of hepatitis B e-antigen: the incidence investigation teams and others. N Eng J Med 1997;336:178–84.
76. Hennekens CH. Hemodialysis-associated hepatitis: an outbreak among hospital personnel. JAMA 1973;225:407–8.
77. Snydman DR, Bryan JA, Macon EJ, et al. Hemodialysis-associated hepatitis: a report of an epidemic with further evidence on mechanisms of transmission. Am J Epidemiol 1976;104:563–70.
78. Garibaldi RA, Forrest JN, Bryan JA, et al. Hemodialysis-associated hepatitis. JAMA 1973;225:384–9.
79. Alter MJ. The epidemiology of acute and chronic hepatitis C. Clin Liver Dis 1997;1:559–68.
80. Lanphear BP, Linnemann CC Jr, Cannon CG, et al. Hepatitis C virus infection in healthcare workers: risk of exposure and infection. Infect Control Hosp Epidemiol 1994;15:745–50.

81. Puro V, Petrosillo N, Ippolito G. Italian study group on occupational risk of HIV and other bloodborne infections. Risk of hepatitis C seroconversion after occupational exposure in health care workers. Am J Infect Control 1995;23:273–7.
82. Mitsui T, Iwano K, Masuko K, et al. Hepatitis C virus infection in medical personnel after needlestick accident. Hepatology 1992;16:1109–14.
83. Sartori M, La Terra G, Aglietta M, et al. Transmission of hepatitis C via blood splash into conjunctiva [letter]. Scand J Infect Dis 1993;25:270–1.
84. Ippolito G, Puro V, Petrosillo N, et al. Simultaneous infection with HIV and hepatitis C virus following occupational conjunctival blood exposure [letter]. JAMA 1998; 280:28.
85. Davis GL, Lau JYN, Urdea MS, et al. Quantitative detection of hepatitis C virus RNA with a solid-phase signal amplification method: definition of optimal conditions for specimen collection and clinical application in interferon-treated patients. Hepatology 1994;19:1337–41.
86. Garner JS. Hospital Infection Control Practices Advisory Committee. Guideline for isolation precautions in hospitals. Infect Control Hosp Epidemiol 1996;17: 54–80.

Health Care–Associated Hepatitis B and C Viruses: Legal Aspects

Mary Anne Bobinski, BA, JD, LLM

KEYWORDS

- Legal • Law • Liability • Hepatitis
- Occupational transmission • Nosocomial infection

The hepatitis B virus (HBV) "is transmitted through percutaneous or mucosal exposure to infectious blood or body fluids."[1] Chronic HBV infection is associated with "cirrhosis of the liver, liver cancer, liver failure, and death."[1] A vaccine is available to prevent HBV infection. The immunization strategy for unvaccinated persons focuses on universal vaccination for infants; routine vaccination of children and adolescents; universal vaccination "[i]n settings in which a high proportion of persons are likely to be at risk for HBV infection"; and routine vaccination for adults with risk factors in other settings.[1] The probability of infection postexposure can be reduced by the timely use of postexposure prophylaxis.[1]

The hepatitis C virus (HCV) is "transmitted primarily through large or repeated direct percutaneous exposures to blood."[2] For most infected persons, HCV infection becomes chronic. Chronic infection is associated with chronic liver disease, cirrhosis, liver cancer, and death.[2] There is no vaccine for HCV and no effective postexposure prophylaxis.[2,3] Hepatitis C "is the most common bloodborne infection in the United States"; there are "an estimated 3.2 million chronically infected persons."[3]

Hepatitis B and C present risks in health care environments because of the prevalence of exposure to blood or other contaminated substances under conditions likely to facilitate transmission of the viruses from infected to uninfected persons.[1,2] Data from the United States indicate that only a small percentage of the estimated 46,000 new cases of hepatitis B infection occurring in 2006 arose in health care settings: "The proportion of persons who reported receiving hemodialysis or a blood transfusion (both of which historically were major sources of infection) or having had occupational exposure to blood was low (0.2%, 0.6%, and 0.5%, respectively)."[3] There were an estimated 19,000 new HCV infections in 2006.[3] Sixteen percent of persons newly infected with HCV reported having had surgery and "1.5% reported occupational exposure to blood."[3] Recent reports indicate continuing concern about the transmission of HCV in hemodialysis[4–6] and in oncology care.[7]

Faculty of Law, University of British Columbia, 1822 East Mall, Vancouver, British Columbia V6T 1Z1, Canada
E-mail address: bobinski@law.ubc.ca

Clin Liver Dis 14 (2010) 105–117
doi:10.1016/j.cld.2009.11.002
1089-3261/10/$ – see front matter © 2010 Elsevier Inc. All rights reserved.

liver.theclinics.com

The risk of hepatitis B and C transmission in health care settings has generated considerable attention within the legal system. This article begins with an overview of the relevant sources of law and then explores legal duties and liability arising from two major categories of risk: occupational risks to health care providers and health care–associated risks to patients and other third parties.

OVERVIEW OF SOURCES OF LAW

One dramatic difference between law and medicine is that legal rules vary from jurisdiction to jurisdiction, whereas the basic principles of medicine and disease remain constant around the world. This presents a bit of a challenge for readers interested in learning more about the legal aspects of hepatitis transmission in health care settings, because the specific governing legal rules vary depending on the location of the concern. In addition, the law is always changing, whether through new legislation, new regulations, new court decisions, or some combination of each. A single article cannot hope to convey the nuances of each jurisdiction's rules. This article does not constitute legal advice and the reader is responsible for seeking specific legal advice from appropriate persons whenever confronting questions about legal responsibilities and consequences.

This article focuses on broad categories of laws, using examples drawn from specific legislation and cases where appropriate. Both the United States and Canada have mixed forms of government with legal rules emanating from the federal level and the state or provincial level. There are many possible sources of legal rules relevant to the problems of hepatitis transmission, ranging from specific legislation governing occupational safety matters to common law tort obligations to act with reasonable care to protect others from the transmission of disease. Most examples are drawn from the United States, where the combination of greater population size and greater focus on liability has resulted in more legislative and judicial activity.

This article divides the legal aspects of health care–associated hepatitis transmission into two broad categories: the legal obligations related to the prevention of transmission and the scope of liability for health care–associated exposure to HBV and HCV. These two categories are closely related given that the violation of legal obligations designed to prevent transmission often give rise to liability for any resulting exposure to these viruses. At the same time, separating the discussion of standards and liability allows the reader to focus on the role of law in establishing standards of care as a topic separate from the special issues related to liability for violations of those standards. The analysis of legal obligations and liabilities includes specific references to the similarities and differences between the ways the legal system treats the risks of HBV and HCV for health care providers as compared with health care patients.

LEGAL STANDARDS RELATING TO THE PREVENTION OF TRANSMISSION

The legal standards relating to the prevention of HBV and HCV transmission are complex. More than in many other areas of medical practice, the risks of HBV and HCV have given rise to standards of care that have been specifically written into relatively detailed legislative and regulatory requirements by national, state, or provincial regulators. The area is also complex because the legal requirements or constraints on medical practice arise in a number of different areas. This article reviews five major areas where legal standard or obligations have been developed that require health care providers to take or to refrain from taking specific measures to reduce the risk of HBV or HCV transmission: (1) requirements for screening and testing of blood, organs, and tissue; (2) the implementation of universal or general precautions including HBV vaccination for health care workers; (3) the rules governing pre-exposure testing and confidentiality for patients and providers; (4) the implementation of practice restrictions for certain HBV-infected health care providers; and (5) the rules governing postexposure prophylaxis.

Screening Requirements

HBV and HCV are readily transmitted through infected materials, such as through blood donations. The legal duty to take measures to prevent transmission has a number of sources. In part because many states in the United States have "blood shield" laws barring common law products liability claims,[8] these duties have been established through regular negligence principles or through specific standards, statutes, and regulations applicable to different types of infectious biologic materials.

From a negligence standpoint, persons involved in the collection of blood, organs, or other bodily substances meant for uses that could involve the risk of HBV and HCV infection have a duty to take reasonable precautions to reduce or eliminate the risk under common law tort rules.[8-10] The specific measures to be taken vary based on the knowledge of the risk and the ability to adopt policies and practices likely to reduce the harm. Before the development of a test for HBV infection, for example, blood banking organizations began to screen donors for risk factors. The blood banks also had a duty to use testing once it became feasible to do so.

The general legal requirement to implement HBV and HCV screening is now well-established, yet the specific legal source of the obligation varies depending on the type of infectious biologic material. Private accreditation standards,[11] federal regulations,[12] and state law[13] apply to a wide range of entities involved with collecting and transferring potentially infectious materials.

The federal regulations require covered entities to implement HBV and HCV testing for blood or blood components intended for certain uses.[12] Donors with positive screening test results are to be notified. The federal rules also implement "look back" procedures for persons who may have previously received blood or blood products from donors testing positive for HCV.[12]

California provides one example of state legislation.[13] The California statute requires testing donors of tissues intended for transfer to another person for a variety of infections, including HBV and HCV.[13] The legislation provides that "No tissues shall be transferred into the body of another person by means of transplantation, unless the donor of the tissues has been screened and found nonreactive by laboratory tests for evidence of infection with . . . agents of viral hepatitis (HBV and HCV)" with some specific exceptions (eg, sperm donations with appropriate consent and vaccination for HBV, defined emergencies, or situations in which the recipient is less likely to be injured by the virus because of previous infection or the likelihood that the disease will not manifest during the recipient's expected lifespan).[13]

Despite the web of regulation, commentators have expressed concern about the relative absence of standards in some areas as advances in medicine created new areas of possible exposure. Human tissue banks have been a particular area of concern.[14] The US Food and Drug Administration issued new rules regarding tissue banking and transplantation in 2007.[15] The regulations make clear that donor specimens must be tested for HBV and HCV and that donors should be screened for risk factors and clinical evidence of HBV and HCV.[15] The regulations also establish detailed recordkeeping requirements.[15]

The Legal Duty to Implement Universal or Standard Precautions

The implementation of universal or standard precautions to prevent the transmission of bloodborne infections is an excellent example of the unusually close relationship between developments in medical practice and the imposition of legal requirements. Generally speaking, medical practice is understood to be particularly within the knowledge and expertise of health care providers. Traditional medical malpractice rules simply require that physicians and other health care providers observe the "standard of care," that they take the actions that a reasonable physician, other professional, or health care institution would take to protect patients and health care workers from the risk of HBV and HCV transmission.[16,17] The standard of care with respect to reducing the risk of health care–associated transmission of HBV and HCV is established by expert testimony in a lawsuit brought by an injured person; the medical experts rely on their own expertise but reference specific practice standards or guidelines issued by the US Centers for Disease Control and Prevention (CDC).[18,19]

The traditional medical malpractice approach has been aggressively supplemented by various forms of legislation and regulation establishing particular standards to reduce the risks of bloodborne pathogens including HBV and HCV. In the late 1980s, for example, federal legislation in the United States required the CDC to develop and promulgate standards to reduce the risk of transmission of HIV to health care workers; the guidelines issued by the CDC also specifically incorporated provisions to reduce the risks associated with HBV.[19] The federal legislation required the federal Department of Labor to use the guidelines in developing workplace safety regulations, commonly known as the "OSHA bloodborne pathogen rule," which was first promulgated in 1991.[20,21] Infection control procedures have continued to become more comprehensive in their approach to risk reduction for a wide variety of diseases; they are also available for a wide range of practice settings.[22–24] Legislative bodies and administrative agencies have responded with updated requirements.[25] States and provinces have also adopted legislation and regulations designed to reduce the risk of HBV and HCV transmission along with other risks, often through professional or institutional licensure and workplace safety rules.[19,26,27]

The United States bloodborne pathogen rule and similar legal standards adopted by states or at the provincial level in Canada involve several types of measures designed to reduce the risk of transmission. Generally, health care entities are required (1) to develop exposure control plans to minimize or eliminate the exposure of employees to bloodborne pathogens and to provide adequate training to employees to carry out the plan; (2) to implement engineering and work practice controls designed to eliminate or minimize exposure including the use of personal protective equipment and specific practices and equipment to prevent injury by needles and other sharps; (3) to implement free and voluntary HBV vaccination and postexposure evaluation and prophylactic treatment; and (4) to carry out specific recordkeeping requirements about exposure incidents.[21,26]

The federal occupational safety and health rules (or similar approved state occupational standards) create legal duties for covered health care employers, such as hospitals and physician offices.[21] The occupational safety rules are enforced through inspections and fines.[28,29] Failure to comply with infection control standards can also result in disciplinary action against individual health care providers under licensure codes.[30]

Pre-exposure Testing and Confidentiality for Patients

HBV and HCV are transmitted by infected persons. This raises questions about whether testing can be used to identify infected patients and whether any available information about HBV and HCV infection can be disclosed to others who might come into contact with infected blood or body fluids.

The general presumption implicit in the use of standard precautions is that the risk of HBV and HCV transmission can best be reduced by exercising the required level of care with all patients rather than attempting to exercise care only with those patients known to have a bloodborne pathogen.[24] Specific knowledge of a patient's HBV and HCV status is not routinely necessary because health care providers exercise the same level of care for all patients. Patients generally have a legal right to control their own health care, including the decision of whether or not to be tested for hepatitis.[16] A patient typically does not have a duty to inform his or her health care provider of the risk the patient may pose because of HBV and HCV infection.[31] Moreover, health care entities and health care personnel have a legal duty to maintain the confidentiality of patient information.[16,32,33] This duty arises from a variety of common law and legislative sources, including the federal Privacy Rule adopted under the Health Insurance Portability and Accountability Act in the United States.[32–34]

These general principles do not reflect the reality of health care settings, where information about patients' HBV and HCV status may be routinely available in patients' medical records. Patients typically sign a general consent to care and treatment within health care facilities that is often broad enough to cover testing for HBV and HCV where necessary for the patient's care and treatment. The Health Insurance Portability and Accountability Act Privacy Rule permits covered health care entities to use or to disclose otherwise confidential health care information about patients "for its own treatment . . . or health care operations."[31] Health care providers may have access to patients' HBV and HCV status.

There is conflicting case law on whether health care providers can refuse to provide care to patients in some limited set of circumstances where there might be a more significant risk of infection despite the use of standard or even specialized precautions. In one case, a person with a disability who was infected with HBV challenged his exclusion from a residential rehabilitation center arguing that the exclusion constituted impermissible discrimination based on disability.[35] A lower court decided that the patient was "qualified" to participate in the residential treatment program because the risk of HBV transmission could be reduced by requiring selected employees to undergo HBV vaccination.[35] The federal court of appeals overturned this decision, finding that the significant risk of transmission in the plaintiff's particular case could only be eliminated through a more expensive inoculation program.[35] A more recent US Supreme Court case makes clear, however, that health care providers cannot refuse to provide care for persons with contagious diseases merely because of a good-faith personal risk assessment.[36] Instead, the risk assessment must be based on medical or other objective evidence.[36] This requirement is unlikely to be met in cases involving health care for persons infected by HBV and HCV given the existing public health guidance emphasizing the reduction of risk through the measures identified in the bloodborne pathogen rule and the use of standard precautions rather than refusal of care.[21,24]

Special Considerations for HBV- or HCV-Infected Providers

The discovery of HIV and public concern about the risk of HIV transmission from infected health care providers to their patients indirectly led to greater attention for the risks presented by HBV-infected providers to their patients. In 1991, the CDC issued guidelines designed to prevent transmission of HIV and HBV from health care workers to patients.[37]

The CDC guidelines, which Congress required states to implement as a condition of receiving certain federal funding, had several principles.[38] The CDC recommended that all health care workers use universal precautions. No practice restrictions were necessary for HBV-infected health care workers "who perform invasive procedures not identified as exposure-prone, provided the infected health care workers (HCWs) practice recommended surgical or dental technique and comply with universal precautions and current recommendations for sterilization/disinfection."[37] The CDC recommended, however, that health care organizations and entities identify "exposure-prone" invasive procedures carrying a heightened risk of exposure for patients. Health care workers who performed these exposure-prone procedures "who do not have serologic evidence of immunity to HBV from vaccination or from previous infection should know their hepatitis B surface antigen (HBsAG) status and, if that is positive, should also know their hepatitis B e antigen (HBeAG) status."[37] Health care workers infected with HBV who are hepatitis B e antigen positive "should not perform exposure-prone procedures unless they have sought counsel from an expert review panel and been advised under what circumstances, if any, they may continue to perform these procedures."[37] The CDC indicated that prospective patients should be "notifyi[ed]… of the health care workers' seropositivity before they undergo exposure-prone invasive procedures."[37] The guidelines emphasized voluntary rather than mandatory testing for health care workers.[37]

The CDC guidelines were widely adopted into United States law with some variations in matters, such as the health care provider's duty to disclose.[38,39] Canada seems to have accepted the broad outlines of the CDC approach as a standard of practice, although implementation at the provincial level may not be uniform.[40,41]

Commentators note the relatively low risks of transmission, the failure of medical organizations to develop a consensus around the definition of exposure-prone procedures, and the asymmetric disclosure obligation suggested for health care workers.[38–40,42] Mandatory disclosure rules are often deemed the equivalent of restrictions on practice given public fears about the risks of transmission.[43]

The original CDC guidelines did not address health care workers infected by HCV. In 1998, the CDC indicated that there was insufficient evidence of risk to justify practice restrictions for HCV-infected health care workers.[2] Some groups have emphasized the need to move forward with evidence-based approaches to implementing restrictions on practice for health care workers infected with HBV and HCV.[39,42,44]

Postexposure Testing and Prophylaxis

The United States bloodborne pathogen rule establishes procedures for postexposure testing and prophylaxis.[21] Employers are to give employees free access to "HBV vaccine and vaccination series and post-exposure evaluation and follow-up, including prophylaxis."[21] Courts have affirmed that the rule requires employers to compensate employees for time spent receiving treatment and for travel expenses.[45]

One significant issue has been whether health care workers exposed to the blood or body fluids of a patient could seek to have the "source" tested for HBV and HCV or other transmissible conditions. The bloodborne pathogen rule provides that the employee should be provided with "[i]dentification and documentation of the source individual, unless the employer can establish that identification is infeasible or prohibited by state or local law."[21] Further, the source individual's blood shall be tested as soon as feasible and after consent is obtained to determine HBV infectivity. If consent is not obtained, the employer shall establish that legally required consent cannot be obtained. When the source individual's consent is not required by law, the source individual's blood, if available, shall be tested and the results documented.[21]

The bloodborne pathogen rule ties directly to state laws regarding testing and confidentiality. Legislation in various states and provinces permits specific persons, typically including at least some emergency responders and health care providers, to seek testing of source individuals.[40,46,47] Guidelines for postexposure testing for HCV infection have also been developed, despite the lack of a HCV vaccine or a well-documented postexposure prophylactic treatment.[22,44]

LIABILITY ASSOCIATED WITH EXPOSURE AND TRANSMISSION

This section turns to the important issue of liability: when and how have defendants been held liable for exposure to or transmission of HBV and HCV in health care settings? There are two main forms of liability for HBV and HCV exposure: tort liability and workers' compensation.

Tort Liability

Tort duties typically arise from the common law, from the decisions of judges and juries in a particular jurisdiction finding that a particular defendant breached a duty to the plaintiff and that breach caused a legally compensable injury. There are two main forms of tort liability potentially relevant to claims involving the transmission of HBV and HCV in health care settings: strict liability and negligence. Under strict liability, manufacturers or sellers of products can be held liable for injuries caused by defective products. Under negligence, health care providers or other defendants can be held liable for damages caused by breaching the duty to use reasonable care to protect patients or others from the risk of HIV infection. Strict liability claims are generally easier for plaintiffs to bring because they often do not require proof that the defendant acted carelessly or unreasonably in failing to prevent transmission. Instead, the plaintiff need only prove that a product was defective and unreasonably dangerous.[16,17]

Blood transfusion and other uses of human tissue

HBV and HCV infection can be transmitted through blood transfusion and the use of other types of infected human tissues. One important initial question is whether strict liability applies to blood transfusions and to the use of human tissue in health care settings. Plaintiffs are more likely to be successful in bringing claims for damages against health care defendants under strict liability. Many jurisdictions have enacted specific "blood shield" statutes, however, that prohibit the use of strict liability or implied warranties in cases involving blood, blood products, and in some jurisdictions other types of human tissue.[8-10] In these jurisdictions, blood transfusions are considered "services" rather than "products" and plaintiffs are not able to bring claims for strict liability for the sale of defective and unreasonably dangerous products. Plaintiffs in these jurisdictions may be restricted from bringing damage claims against some parties in the blood collection and distribution process (eg, against donors) or may be required to bring any claim under negligence theory rather than strict liability.[8-10]

Blood shield legislation was designed to support continued use of blood and blood products, which were viewed as being socially valuable and yet incapable of being rendered completely safe. The blood shield laws are a form of protection: blood banking and blood products continue to be available at reasonable cost because their producers are not required to pay the costs of many injuries caused by these important products. Blood shield statutes make it more likely that the costs of injuries associated with the use of blood are borne by injured individuals rather than by all those who use (and pay for) blood products, as would be the case if the prices of blood products were adjusted to include the costs of compensating persons injured by those products.

Although negligence claims are more difficult that strict liability claims, plaintiffs have nonetheless been successful in seeking damages from some blood banking entities and health care providers for failing to use due care to prevent transmission of HBV and HCV.[8-10] Blood banking organizations are often held to a "professional" standard of care that requires the use of experts and at least some consideration of whether the defendants were following reasonable industry practices.[9,10] Some successful claims have been based on the failure of defendants to use reasonably available methods, such as donor screening or testing, to prevent the use of infected blood or blood products.[9] Other claims involve the failure of health care provider defendants to obtain appropriate informed consent from patients regarding the risks associated with the use of blood or other potentially infectious materials.[9] It is important to note that the plaintiff must be able to demonstrate that the defendant's breach of the standard of care actually caused the harm and that the plaintiff would more likely than not have avoided infection had the defendant exercised the required level of care.[48] The difficulties of bringing individual negligence actions are sometimes avoided by class actions or special compensation funds established by governments. Canada established a special compensation fund for hemophiliacs infected by HCV.[49]

Transmission in health care settings

There is a risk of HBV and HCV transmission in health care settings through exposure of patients, providers, or even visitors to infected body fluids under circumstances where transmission is possible (eg, through a needle stick, blood splash, or exposure to an open wound). Transmission clearly is possible in surgery but has also been found in outpatient settings,[50] in hemodialysis centers,[4-6] and through oncology care.[7] Risky practices have continued, despite the development of detailed guidance about the changes in practices necessary to reduce the risk of transmission.[24,51,52] Two cases provide examples of some of the typical issues in tort claims arising from the transmission of HBV and HCV in health care settings.

In *Bouchard et al v Savoie*,[53] a New Brunswick court considered a claim brought by a surgeon against a hospital. The plaintiff surgeon performed an operation on a patient known to be infected with HBV; "[a]ll personnel involved in the operation were duly warned, and elaborate precautionary measures were taken."[53] The surgeon "sustained a 'needle stick' from a used syringe which... had seemingly not been retrieved from the area of the operation from the scrub nurse."[53] The surgeon became infected by HBV and suffered injuries, such as illness and lost income. The surgeon sought to hold the nurse and the nurse's employing hospital liable for these losses. The hospital argued in defense that the surgeon had caused the injury by failing to use proper procedures to remove the syringe from the field of the operation and that the physician effectively controlled the actions of the defendant nurse during surgery. The appellate court upheld the trial court's determination that both the plaintiff and defendant contributed to the injuries and affirmed most aspects of a damage award to the physician for a percentage of his claimed losses. The case is useful because it demonstrates the potential for liability even in cases where the person infected with HBV and HCV arguably was partially responsible for his or her injury.

In *Hardiman v Davita Inc*, the court considered a claim brought by a hemodialysis patient against a hemodialysis center based on the alleged transmission of HBV.[54] The plaintiff argued that he had acquired HBV infection from the dialysis center because of the center's lack of care in failing to immunize him and in failing to quarantine patients infected with HBV.[54] The magistrate considered a variety of arguments revolving around whether the plaintiff had provided sufficient expert evidence about the likely source of the HBV to permit the case to move forward. The court found that the plaintiff's expert was qualified to testify and that the plaintiff had presented sufficient evidence to justify allowing his case to move forward. The case focuses on the key role of expert evidence in these cases.

Special topic: damages

Defendants in tort claims can be required to compensate plaintiffs for their injuries. Typical injuries in cases of HBV and HCV transmission include pain and suffering, disability, lost income, and medical costs. Because the natural course of hepatitis infection can vary from person to person, it is not always possible for the plaintiff to present the required proof demonstrating that it is more likely than not that he or she will experience some forms of damages.

Cases of exposure to HBV and HCV also raise a more controversial type of damage in cases where the virus is not actually transmitted. In these cases, plaintiffs seem to recover for the emotional distress or fear that they experience between the exposure incident and the final determination that transmission did not occur. Many cases have arisen in health care settings after needle sticks or other injuries. "Look back" programs, such as those notifying patients that they have received care from an infected health care worker or that they have received blood or tissue from a donor who later tested positive for HCV,[12] can create significant anxiety for individuals. If the recipients of these notifications believe that the underlying exposure incident arose because of negligence, then a claim for emotional distress damages may result. A number of courts have confronted these disease "phobia" claims, often in the context of HIV but also with respect to hepatitis.[55,56] The legal issues and principles are the same for both diseases.

Courts confronted with disease phobia claims initially struggled to determine when and how to compensate persons who sought damages for the fear that transmission might have occurred. Although there is variation across jurisdictions, the emerging majority approach seems to require proof of actual exposure to support a claim for negligent infliction of emotional distress.[55] "Actual exposure" typically means proof both that the "source" individual was infected with the disease and that there was an exposure incident capable of transmitting the virus even though transmission did not actually occur.[55]

In *Russaw v Martin et al*,[56] for example, a syringe that had been used to administer medication to a patient fell out of the pocket of a nurse and became stuck in the plaintiff's leg. The nurse initially indicated the needle was clean but then revealed that it was used. The plaintiff and the source patient both consented to hepatitis and HIV testing with negative results. The plaintiff and her husband also tested negative several times over the next few months.[56] The defendant argued that the needle never had come into contact with the source patient's bodily fluids. The Georgia appeals court rejected the plaintiff's claim: "Because the Russaws offered no evidence of actual exposure to HIV or AIDS or hepatitis and no evidence of a channel of communication of disease, we hold that their recovery for fear and mental anguish is per se unreasonable as a matter of law."[56] The case demonstrates the circumstances in which fear of hepatitis claims can arise and the requirements of the actual exposure rule.

Workers' Compensation

Workers' compensation laws provide a mechanism for injured workers to receive compensation for their injuries without the expense and uncertainty of negligence actions. The benefit for injured workers is matched by the benefit to employers because the level of compensation under workers' compensation is lower than what might have been awarded in a successful negligence suit. Legislation typically requires injured workers to bring claims under workers' compensation schemes rather than through the tort system in most cases.

Workers' compensation provides a possible avenue for recovery for employees, such as nurses or other caregivers, who are infected by HBV and HCV transmission in health care settings. Many health care employees in positions carrying a risk for hepatitis transmission are now undergoing vaccination for HBV and postexposure prophylaxis is available. HCV therefore is an increasingly important workers' compensation issue. Nonemployees, such as nonemployee physicians, are not eligible for workers' compensation.[53] The central issue in workers' compensation claims involving HBV and HCV is whether the disease was acquired through occupational or nonoccupational exposure. Some jurisdictions have issued legislative or administrative guidelines establishing the review criteria and likely disposition of HBV and HCV claims in health care settings.[57] Disputes over workers' compensation typically involve uncertainty about when transmission occurred and whether it occurred in or out of the workplace.[58] The workers' compensation laws are often interpreted to provide extra protections for workers.

FUTURE LEGAL CONSIDERATIONS

This article demonstrates the important role law plays in establishing the standards and procedures used to reduce the risk of HBV and HCV transmission in health care settings and the importance of law in providing compensation for injured persons. The close connection between medical developments and legal requirements is likely to continue in the years ahead.

REFERENCES

1. Mast E, Weinbaum CM, Fiore AE, et al. A comprehensive immunization strategy to eliminate transmission of hepatitis B virus infection in the United States, recommendations of the Advisory Committee on Immunization Practices (ACIP). Part II: immunization of adults. MMWR Recomm Rep 2006;55(RR-16):1–33.
2. Centers for Disease Control and Prevention. Recommendations for prevention and control of hepatitis C virus (HCV) infection and HCV-related chronic disease. MMWR Recomm Rep 1998;47(RR-19):1–39.
3. Wasley A, Grytdal S, Gallagher K. Surveillance for acute viral hepatitis—United States. MMWR Surveill Summ 2006;57(SS-2):1–24.
4. Hepatitis C. Virus transmission at an outpatient hemodialysis unit—New York, 2001–2008. MMWR Morb Mortal Wkly Rep 2009;58(8):189–94.
5. Agarwal SK, Dash SC, Gupta S, et al. Hepatitis C virus infection in haemodialysis: the no-isolation policy should not be generalized. Nephron Clin Pract 2009; 111(2):c133–40.
6. Alavaian SM. A shield against a monster: hepatitis C in hemodialysis patients. World J Gastroenterol 2009;15(6):641–6.
7. Sepkowitz K. Risk to cancer patients from nosocomial hepatitis C virus. Infect Control Hosp Epidemiol 2004;25:599–602.

8. Kussmann P. Validity, construction, and application of blood shield statutes. American Law Reports 2000;75(5):229 (electronically supplemented through 2009).
9. Zitter JM. Liability of hospital, physician, or other individual medical practitioner for injury or death resulting from blood transfusion. American Law Reports 1983;20(4):136 (electronically supplemented through 2009).
10. Zitter JM. Liability of blood supplier or donor for injury or death resulting from blood transfusion. American Law Reports 1983;24:508 (electronically supplemented through 2009).
11. AABB, Accreditation. Available at: http://www.aabb.org/Content/Accreditation/accreditation.htm. Accessed April 25, 2009. (AABB was formerly known as the American Association of Blood Banks).
12. U.S. Food and Drug Administration, Test requirements. 21 Code of Federal Regulations. §610.40–.48 & 630.6; 2009.
13. Transplantation of tissues; screening tests for infectious diseases of donors; regulations; prohibition of use of infected tissues. Cal Health and Safety Code Ann §1644.5; 2009. Available at: http://www.law.cornell.edu/citation/2-300.htm.
14. Buck LA. Regulating human tissue banks. St Thomas Law Rev 2007;20: 121–53.
15. U.S. Food and Drug Administration. Human tissue intended for transplantation. 21 Code of Federal Regulations. §1270.1–.43; 2009.
16. Hall MA, Bobinski MA, Orentlicher D. Health care law and ethics. 7th edition. New York: Aspen Publishers; 2007. p. 173–272, 313–6.
17. Dickens B. Medical negligence. In: Downie J, Caulfield T, Flood CM, editors. Canadian health law and policy. 3rd edition. LexisNexis (Canada): Markham; 2007. p. 101–34.
18. Centers for Disease Control. Perspectives in disease prevention and health promotion update: universal precautions for prevention of transmission of human immunodeficiency virus, and other bloodborne pathogens in health-care settings. MMWR Morb Mortal Wkly Rep 1988;37(24):377–88.
19. Centers for Disease Control. Guidelines for prevention of transmission of human immunodeficiency virus and hepatitis B virus to health-care and public-safety workers a response to P.L. 100-607 The Health Omnibus Programs Extension Act of 1988. MMWR Morb Mortal Wkly Rep 1989;38(S-6):3–37.
20. Occupational safety and health administration, occupational exposure to bloodborne pathogens: final rule. Fed Regist. 1991;56:64175–82.
21. Bloodborne pathogens rule. 29 Code of Federal Regulations. §1910.1030; 2009.
22. Centers for Disease Control and Prevention. Updated U.S. public health service guidelines for the management of occupational exposures to HBV, HCV, and HIV and recommendations for postexposure prophylaxis. MMWR Recomm Rep 2001; 50(RR-11):1–52.
23. Kohn WG, Collins AS, Cleveland JL, et al. Guidelines for infection control in dental health-care settings—2003. MMWR Recomm Rep 2003;52(RR-17): 1–66.
24. Siegel J.D. Rhinehart E. Jackson M. 2007 Guideline for isolation precautions: preventing transmission of infectious agents in healthcare settings. 2007. Available at: http://www.cdc.gov/ncidod/dhqp/pdf/guidelines/Isolation2007.pdf. Accessed April 25, 2009.
25. Needlestick Safety and Prevention Act. Public Law 106-430, 106th Congress, 2nd Sess, 114 STAT. 1901 (2000). Available at: http://www.gpoaccess.gov/plaws/index.html.

26. Province of British Columbia, WorkSafeBC. Occupational health and safety regulation. 6.33–36.40, unofficial version. Available at: http://www2.worksafebc.com/publications/OHSRegulation/Part6.asp#SectionNumber:6.33. Accessed March 22, 2009.

27. National Institute for Occupational Safety and Health, U.S. Centers for Disease Control and Prevention. Overview of state needle safety legislation. Available at: http://www.cdc.gov/niosh/topics/bbp/ndl-law.html. Accessed April 26, 2009.

28. Cuming RG, Rocco RS, McEachern AG. Improving compliance with occupational safety and health administration standards. AORN J 2008;87(2):347–56.

29. U.S. Occupational Safety and Health Administration. Enforcement procedures for the occupational exposure to bloodborne pathogens (CPL 02-02-069, 2001). Available at: http://www.osha.gov/pls/oshaweb/owadisp.show_document?p_table=DIRECTIVES&p_id=2570. Accessed April 11, 2009.

30. Rosov v Maryland state board of dental examiners, 877 A.2d 1111 (Md. App. 2005). Available at: http://en.wikipedia.org/wiki/Atlantic_Reporter and http://west.thomson.com/productdetail/1454/22011606/productdetail.aspx.

31. Oddi AS. Reverse informed consent: the unreasonably dangerous patient. Vanderbilt Law Rev 1992;46:1417–83 (arguing that such a duty should be created).

32. Health Insurance Portability and Accountability Act of 1996 Privacy Rule, 45 Code of Federal Regulations. §§160.101–.552, 164.102–.106, 164.500–.534 (2009).

33. Office of Civil Rights, U.S. Department Health and Human Services. Privacy rule. Available at: http://www.hhs.gov/ocr/privacy/hipaa/administrative/privacyrule/index.html. Accessed April 26, 2009.

34. Snavely v AMISUB of South Carolina, Inc, 665 S.E.2d 222 (S.C. App. 2008). (patient unsuccessful in bringing breach of confidentiality action against health care provider in case involving disclosure of HBV status). Available at: http://en.wikipedia.org/wiki/South_Eastern_Reporter.

35. Kohl v Woodhaven Learning Center, 865 F.2d 930 (8th Cir. 1989), cert. denied 493 U.S. 892 (1989). Available at: http://en.wikipedia.org/wiki/Federal_Reporter.

36. Bragdon v Abbott, 524 U.S. 624 (1998). Available at: http://en.wikipedia.org/wiki/Case_citation.

37. Recommendations for preventing transmission of human immunodeficiency virus and hepatitis B virus to patients during exposure-prone invasive procedures. U.S. Centers for Disease Control and Prevention. MMWR Recomm Rep 1991;40(RR08):1–9.

38. Gostin LO. A proposed national policy on health care workers living with HIV/AIDS and other blood-borne pathogens. JAMA 2000;284(15):1965–70.

39. Reitsma AM, Closen ML, Cunningham M, et al. Infected physicians and invasive procedures: safe practice management. Clin Infect Dis 2005;40:1665–72.

40. Bobinski M. HIV/AIDS and public health law. In: Bailey TM, Caulfield T, Ries NM, editors. Public health law and policy in Canada. 2nd edition. LexisNexis (Canada): Markham; 2008. p. 189–245.

41. Public Health Agency of Canada. Information infected health care worker: risk of transmission of bloodborne pathogens. Available at: http://www.phac-aspc.gc.ca/publicat/info/infbbp-eng.php. Accessed April 25, 2009.

42. Perry JL, Pearson MD, Jaffer J. Infected health care workers and patient safety: a double standard. Am J Infect Control 2006;34(5):313–9.

43. Tuboku-Metzger JT, Chiarello L, Sinkowitz-Cochran RL, et al. Public attitudes and opinions toward physicians and dentists infected with bloodborne viruses: results of a national survey. Am J Infect Control 2005;33(5):299–303.

44. Henderson DK. Managing occupational risks for hepatitis C transmission in the health care setting. Clin Microbiol Rev 2003;16(3):546–68.
45. Sec'y of Labor v Beverly Healthcare-Hillview, 541 F.3d 193 (3d Cir. 2008). Available at: http://en.wikipedia.org/wiki/Federal_Reporter.
46. Testing required when health care worker exposed to bloodborne disease. S.C. Code 1976 Ann.§ 44-29-230. Available at: http://www.law.cornell.edu/citation/2-300.htm.
47. Moloughney BW. Transmission and post-exposure management of bloodborne virus infections in the healthcare setting: where are we now? CMAJ 2001;165(4):445–51.
48. Grant v American National Red Cross, 745 A.2d 316 (D.C.App. 2000). Available at: http://en.wikipedia.org/wiki/Atlantic_Reporter and http://west.thomson.com/productdetail/1454/22011606/productdetail.aspx.
49. Angelotta C, McKay JM, Fisher MJ, et al. Legal, financial, and public health consequences of transfusion-transmitted hepatitis C virus in persons with haemophilia. Vox Sang 2007;93:159–65.
50. U.S. Centers for Disease Control and Prevention. Transmission of hepatitis B and C viruses in outpatient settings—New York, Oklahoma, and Nebraska, 2000–2002. MMWR Morb Mortal Wkly Rep 2003;52(38):901–6.
51. CBC News. Thousands face infection risk after syringes reused at Alberta hospital. Monday, October 27, 2008. Available at: http://www.cbc.ca/canada/edmonton/story/2008/10/27/high-prairie.html. Accessed April 27, 2009.
52. AP.U.S. hepatitis campaign warns against reusing plastic syringes. February 6, 2009. Available at: http://www.cbc.ca/health/story/2009/02/05/hepatitis.html. Accessed April 27, 2009.
53. Bouchard et al v Savoie, 26 C.C.L.T 173, 49 N.B.R. (2d) 424, 129 A.P.R. 424 (N.B. App. 1983). Available at: http://en.wikipedia.org/wiki/Case_citation.
54. Hardiman v Davita, Inc, 2007 WL 1395568 (N.D. Ind.). Available at: http://en.wikipedia.org/wiki/westlaw and http://www.law.cornell.edu/citation/2-200.htm#2-200.
55. Simmons KC. Recovery for emotional distress based on fear of contracting HIV/AIDS. American Law Reports 1998;59(5):535 (electronic version supplemented though 2009).
56. Russaw v Martin et al, 472 S.E.2d 508 (Ga. App. 1996). Available at: http://en.wikipedia.org/wiki/South_Eastern_Reporter.
57. Worksafe BC [British Columbia, Canada], backgrounder, adjudication of HIV and hepatitis B and C exposure claims (February 2006). Available at: http://www2.worksafebc.com/PDFs/Healthcare/Backgrounder_Adj_HIV_HepBC.pdf. Accessed April 29, 2009.
58. Sfikas PM. Workers' compensation and hepatitis C: if an employee contracted the disease while working for another dentist, could you be required to pay compensation? That depends on the circumstances. J Am Dent Assoc 2000;131:1351–3.

Infection Control Guidelines for Prevention of Health Care–Associated Transmission of Hepatitis B and C Viruses

Angela Michelin, MPH, David K. Henderson, MD*

KEYWORDS

• Viral hepatitis • Bloodborne hepatitis infection
• Hepatitis transmission • Occupational medicine

OVERVIEW OF HEALTH CARE–ASSOCIATED TRANSMISSION OF HEPATITIS B AND HEPATITIS C
Patient-to-Provider Transmission

Viral hepatitis was first identified as an occupational hazard for health care workers more than 60 years ago when a blood bank worker was identified as having acquired viral hepatitis as a result of needlestick exposures.[1] Numerous studies subsequently demonstrated that the risk for transmission of hepatitis B virus (HBV) in the health care setting relates directly to exposure to blood. In an elegant study Dienstag and Ryan[2] demonstrated that the prevalence of serologic results suggestive of prior HBV exposure and infection increased as a function of contact with blood, years in a health care occupation, and age. In their study emergency room nurses, pathology staff members, blood bank staff members, laboratory technicians, intravenous teams, and surgical house officers were found to have the highest frequencies of HBV markers. Other studies have reinforced and extended these findings.[3–6] For the past few decades, hepatitis B has been one of the most significant occupational infectious risks for health care providers. With the increasing prevalence of hepatitis C infections around the world, occupational transmission of this flavivirus from infected patients to their providers has also become a significant concern.

NIH Clinical Center, Building 10 Room 6-1480, 10 Center Drive, Bethesda, MD 20892, USA
* Corresponding author.
E-mail address: dhenderson@mail.cc.nih.gov (D.K. Henderson).

Clin Liver Dis 14 (2010) 119–136
doi:10.1016/j.cld.2009.11.005
1089-3261/10/$ – see front matter © 2010 Published by Elsevier Inc.

liver.theclinics.com

Several factors influence the risk for occupational bloodborne hepatitis infection among health care providers, among them: the prevalence of infection among the population served, the infection status of the patients to whom workers are exposed (ie, the source patient's circulating viral burden),[7,8] the types and frequencies of parenteral and mucosal exposures to blood and blood-containing body fluids, and whether the patient or provider has been immunized with the hepatitis B vaccine. Patients who have circulating hepatitis B "e" antigen historically have presented the highest levels of risk for occupational infection[7,8]; however, in the past few years investigators have detected HBV isolates defective in their ability to make "e" antigen (so-called precore mutants of hepatitis B) that often produce infections associated with very high circulating viral burdens.[9] Identification of such strains underscores the importance of measuring the virus directly, as opposed to assaying for surrogate markers for viral burden (eg, "e" antigen). Although not definitively proven, one may reasonably speculate that higher circulating levels of hepatitis C virus (HCV) would also be associated with increased risk for occupational infection.

Numerous anecdotal case reports underscore the risk for transmission of HCV from patients to providers.[10–22] Although blood is the major reservoir for occupational infection, other body substances may represent risks for HCV transmission, particularly if associated with the parenteral route of exposure or with a large inoculum. Nonetheless, to the authors' knowledge, transmission associated with other body substances has not yet been documented, presumably because viral titers in body fluids other than blood are lower than those found in blood. Percutaneous exposures to blood or blood-contaminated devices (eg, needlestick injuries) have traditionally been the most common circumstance resulting in occupational HBV and HCV infections in health care providers. Several cases of infection with both viruses have been associated with mucosal splashes of blood or blood-containing body fluids. HBV is reasonably stable in the health care environment, and environmental contamination has frequently been incriminated in transmission in health care environments, particularly in dialysis units. The risk for transmission of HBV following a parenteral exposure to blood likely depends on a variety of factors, including the source patient's circulating viral burden, the size of the inoculum of blood, the exposed individual's natural immunity and immune responses, and a variety of other factors. Taken together, the risk for transmission of HBV following a percutaneous exposure to blood from a patient known to be HBV infected ranges from 6% to 33% from the older literature, with the higher percentages associated with exposures to blood from patients who are known to be "e" antigen positive (and therefore who have higher circulating viral burdens).[8,23]

Environmental contamination with HCV has been suggested as contributing to transmission in some clinical settings (eg, the hemodialysis)[24–28]; however, to the authors' knowledge HCV transmission solely due to environmental contamination has not been documented definitively. The prevalence of HCV infection among hemodialysis patients varies substantially, with reported rates ranging between 4% and 70%.[28] In a United States survey conducted in 2000, the seroprevalence of HCV infection in the dialysis setting was found to be 1.7% among hemodialysis staff and 8.4% in hemodialysis patients.[29]

Data about the risk for transmission of HCV associated with a discrete exposure are somewhat confusing, primarily because the several studies that have attempted to measure this risk have used a variety of detection systems to document infection (summarized in Ref.[30]). Nonetheless, a reasonable estimate for this risk is between 1% and 2% per exposure,[30] suggesting that the occupational HCV risk is likely to be approximately 10-fold less than the risk associated with an exposure to an "e" antigen positive HBV-infected source.

Patient-to-Patient Transmission

Patient-to-patient transmission of bloodborne pathogens associated with health care processes has been identified as a substantial problem during the past 2 decades, both in the United States and worldwide. Health care–associated patient-to-patient transmission of bloodborne pathogens has become epidemic in some developing countries as a result of: the reuse of blood-contaminated injection needles or syringes without appropriate reprocessing, the inappropriate use of multidose vials, or saline infusions on multiple patients,[31–38] medical error,[39] or the use of other less-than-optimal infection control techniques. Such patient-to-patient transmission has been particularly problematic in pediatric populations. In developed countries, the most important mechanisms of patient-to-patient transmission has been the inappropriate use of multidose vials[31–38] or bags of intravenous saline flush solutions.[24,26,27,30,33,40–46] Outbreaks of both HBV infection[47–51] and HCV infection have been detected. Patient-to-patient transmission of HCV infection has been most frequently detected in hemodialysis.[15,24,26,27,40,52–65] Transmission of both HBV and HCV in the dialysis setting is multifactorial. Suggested risk factors for transmission include: environmental contamination[24–28,66]; contaminated dialysis machines and dialyzers[26,27,67]; inappropriate infection control procedures[24,26,27,52,53,58,68]; treating both infected and noninfected patients in the same dialysis area[52,53,59,62,65]; and understaffing.[62] Particularly in developing countries, health care–associated patient-to-patient transmission of HCV related to faulty injection practices is an increasingly common mechanism of transmission of HCV.[51,69–76] Other devices implicated in the transmission of these pathogens include contaminated spring-loaded finger-stick devices,[44,77] contaminated gynecologic and gynecologic endocrinologic equipment,[78–81] contaminated multidose vials,[35,36,38,79,82,83] contaminated intravenous administration devices,[84] and contaminated endoscopes.[85,86]

Provider-to-Patient Transmission

Provider-to-patient transmission of bloodborne pathogens is the least common mechanism of transmission of these pathogens in the health care setting, and HBV transmission has historically been more frequently detected. A review published in 1994 identified 42 instances of provider-to-patient transmission of hepatitis B.[87] Since 1994, an additional 12 instances of provider-to-patient hepatitis B transmission have been reported[61,74,88–90] (I. Williams, CDC, personal communication, 2007) including transmission from providers who are "e" antigen negative, but who are infected with so-called precore mutants of hepatitis B.[9]

With respect to HCV, several instances of transmission from provider-to-patient have been detected.[80,81,91–103] Of note, the epidemiology of provider-to-patient HCV transmission has been different in Europe and the United States. Most of the European cases involve surgeons who were HCV infected who performed surgical procedures and infected some of their patients, presumably during the course of invasive procedures.[36,81,95,100,101,104–108] In one of the European cases, an anesthesiologist infected a patient during a procedure in which the anesthesiologist endotracheally intubated the patient and provided anesthesia care.[96] Another unusual cluster of 5 cases of HCV involved an anesthesia assistant who was thought to have acquired acute HCV infection as a result of an occupational exposure to an HCV-infected patient in the operating room and then transmitted his infection to 5 of his patients.[109]

Only 4 instances of HCV provider-to-patient transmission of HCV have been detected in the United States. One United States case involved an HCV infected cardiac surgeon who infected as many as 14 of 937 patients over a decade of surgical practice.[46] A major feature of all the remaining instances of provider-to-patient transmission of HCV reported from the United States is injection drug use on the part of the infected provider.[46] In each of these instances investigations identified (or investigators highly suspected) diversion of patients' drugs to health care providers who were using injectable narcotics. Two additional clusters of provider-to-patient HCV infection, one from Spain and the other from Israel, underscore the potential contribution of injecting drug use to the epidemiology of provider-to-patient transmission of HCV infection. In the Spanish cluster an opiate-addicted anesthesiologist infected more than 200 of his patients.[91,110] In the Israeli cluster, an injection-drug-using anesthesiologist infected 33 patients.[102]

With the exception of the cases linked to the diversion of patients' narcotics to injecting drug-using providers, the precise mode of transmission for hepatitis C for the remaining cases is unknown; however, the circumstances surrounding several of the cases suggest that transmission was associated with percutaneous exposures associated with major surgical procedures performed by HCV-infected providers.

PREVENTION STRATEGIES

Overall prevention strategies are summarized in **Box 1**, with the details for each of these interventions discussed in more detail in the text.

Preventing Patient-to-Provider Transmission

Standard precautions

For the past 25 years, United States public health authorities have recommended that health care providers consider all blood and blood-containing body fluids to be potentially infectious,[104,111,112] and that health care providers wear appropriate barriers to prevent contact with blood, other body fluids containing blood, as well as amniotic fluid, semen, vaginal fluid, cerebrospinal fluid, and exudates. In 1996, the Centers for Disease Control and Prevention (CDC) expanded their earlier recommendations to include the adoption of the infection control system now known as Standard Precautions.[113] These precautions apply to *all* patients, irrespective of their known infection statuses. Major components of these guidelines include use of personal protective equipment in appropriate situations, implementation of both work practice controls and engineering controls, and adherence to meticulous standards for the cleaning and reprocessing of patient care equipment.[113] Several studies demonstrated that the use of these precautions resulted in a significant reduction in parenteral occupational exposures for health care workers.[108,114–116]

Work practice and engineering controls

As noted earlier, a major component of Standard Precautions is the implementation of aggressive prevention strategies for percutaneous injuries. Because parenteral exposures are the primary route by which these agents are transmitted in the health care setting, preventing such exposures will prevent the majority of these infections. Components of such a program include avoiding the resheathing of needles, avoiding unnecessary needle and sharp object use (eg, avoiding unnecessary phlebotomies), use of puncture-resistant needle and sharp object disposal containers (located as close as possible to the point of use), using needleless vascular access systems when practical to obtain blood (eg, "ports" and so forth.), and avoiding unnecessary

---

Box 1
Overall prevention strategies

Preventing Patient-to-Provider Transmission

Universal precautions

Hepatitis B vaccination

"Safer" devices (engineering controls)

Work practice controls

Preventing Patient-to-Patient Transmission

Universal precautions

Hepatitis B vaccination

Infection control procedures

Minimizing reuse to the extent possible

Monitor cleaning, disinfection, and sterilization for reusable devices

Avoidance of multidose vials

Preventing Provider-to-Patient Transmission

Universal precautions

Attention to detail of infection control procedures

Work practice controls

Engineering controls/safer devices

Treatment of provider infection

Adherence to guidelines for infected providers

---

placement of intravenous catheters by using needleless or protected needle infusion systems.

The approach to parenteral injury prevention in health care settings in which invasive procedures are conducted follows the same principles of aggressive prevention.[88,117–122] For example, to minimize risk, surgeons and intensivists can use the least invasive approach that provides the optimal outcome, (eg, using adhesive tape, staples, or tissue glue rather than sutures). Use of "no-touch" surgical technique (ie, using instruments, not hands, for retraction of tissue; keeping the hands of additional providers out of the operative field while the surgeon is operating; avoiding passing instruments directly from hand to hand by using an emesis basin or a Mayo stand; and announcing the transfer of sharp instruments before transferring them) is another important component of a parenteral injury prevention program for the operating theater.

Double gloving also provides an additional barrier. Surgical gloves do not provide a barrier to sharp object penetration, but the use of 2 layers of gloves may reduce the volume of blood transferred to the skin and, therefore, decrease the risk for blood-borne pathogen infection. Breakdown in glove integrity may result in contamination of exposed tissue and blood contamination of the provider's hands. In some instances the provider may sustain tissue trauma (eg, needle puncture or shear injury from tying sutures), and the patient may be exposed to the provider's blood or interstitial fluids (discussed later). Double gloving may reduce the risk for these exposures, as is evidenced by the lower prevalence of inner glove perforation during surgical procedures.[105–107,123–130] Others have used reinforcing structures in gloves at the most common glove perforation sites.[117,131–134] Whereas the benefit of double gloving, glove reinforcement, and new glove technology has not been proved definitively, evidence strongly suggests that exposure of the surgeons' hands to blood contamination is dramatically reduced. Double gloving during invasive surgical and obstetric procedures has now become a standard recommendation.[135,136]

The use of work practice controls that have been shown to reduce risks for exposure is another important aspect of Standard Precautions. Modifying procedures that are intrinsically risky (ie, those that are consistently associated with a risk for occupational exposures) to decrease the risk for occupational exposure (and therefore infection) makes implicit sense. The past 3 decades have also seen the development of numerous engineered controls, including resheathing needles, self-blunting needles, and many others. In terms of risks for occupational exposures in the operating theater, the emergency department, and the delivery suite, the suture needle represents the single most important source of these exposures. To address risks associated with suture needles, engineers developed suture needles that have blunted tips, which can replace standard curved suture needles in many clinical settings and minimize the risks associated with standard needles.[137–142] Studies have demonstrated that the use of these needles is effective in preventing intraoperative injuries.[137] In addition, the use of these needles is also associated with a significantly decreased incidence of penetration of surgical gloves, thereby further reducing risk.

Hepatitis B immunization

Hepatitis B immunization of health care workers is a crucial part of any program designed to reduce the risk for health care–associated transmission of HBV. The efficacy of HBV immunization in preventing the transmission of HBV is unquestioned. Immunization can protect the provider and ultimately will protect patients. In the United States, health care workers who have exposure to blood in the health care environment are required either to be immunized with the HBV vaccine or sign a declination.[143]

Preventing Patient-to-Patient Transmission

The prevention of patient-to-patient transmission of bloodborne pathogens relies heavily on strict adherence to the principles of Standard Precautions. Staff education about the principles of Standard Precautions and about infection control principles in general is crucial to the prevention of patient-to-patient transmission of HBV and HCV associated with health care procedures. As noted earlier, many of the documented instances of HBV and HCV patient-to-patient transmission have been associated with less than optimal infection control techniques.[31–38] Minimizing reuse of equipment designed initially for single-patient use, minimizing the use of multidose vials, minimizing the use of saline infusion bags and irrigants for multiple patients, and closely monitoring the efficacy of cleaning, disinfection, and sterilization for reusable devices are all critical aspects of a program designed to reduce the risk for transmission of these hepatitis viruses. The presence of a strong, visible institutional infection control program will have a substantive effect on adherence to these basic principles of infection control. As patient-to-patient transmission of these 2 hepatitis viruses has been disturbingly on the increase, focusing on these principles offers the best opportunity to reduce the risk for health care–associated transmission of hepatitis B and C viruses.

Preventing Provider-to-Patient Transmission

Provider-to-patient transmission of these viruses is the least common mechanism of health care–associated transmission of hepatitis B and C viruses. Strategies designed to decrease the risk for transmission of the agents from providers to their patients have been of 2 general categories: those designed to decrease the likelihood of parenteral exposures that provide the opportunity for recontact of an object contaminated with the blood of an infected provider with her or his patient's tissue, and those designed to restrict the practices of providers who present the highest risk for transmission of these viruses to their patients.

Strategies Designed to Decrease Exposure Risks

With respect to strategies that are designed to decrease the risks for parenteral occupational exposures, many of the strategies discussed earlier in the patient-to-provider and patient-to-patient categories are effective in reducing provider exposures and, therefore, the opportunities for recontact or "bleed-back." Strict adherence to the tenets of Standard Precautions as well as attention to the details of recommended infection control procedures are important principles in reducing risk for exposure. Hepatitis B immunization of providers and patients is another essential principle in decreasing risk for bidirectional transmission of these viruses. Implementation and continuous improvements in work practice and engineered controls, particularly in environments in which invasive procedures are performed, offer additional potential for risk reduction. Many of the safer devices discussed here were designed to prevent providers' parenteral exposures and, if effective, would also decrease the risk for provider-to-patient exposures and infection.

Another important risk reduction strategy is the aggressive treatment of providers found to be infected with these bloodborne viruses. Hepatitis B treatment strategies have been developed over the past decade that can reduce provider's circulating viral burdens, thereby presumably also decreasing the risk for provider-to-patient trans-mission of HBV.[144] HBV monotherapy can render a substantial fraction of previously "e" antigen positive patients "e" antigen negative, with a substantial fraction such patients remaining HBV-DNA negative after 1 year of treatment[144]; however, the development of antiviral resistance is a continued problem. Whether combination therapy will be superior to monotherapy in this setting is at too preliminary a stage to judge. Current therapeutic options for HBV infection only suppress and generally do not eradicate the virus. The evidence base for the therapy for providers infected with HBV is nonexistent, as is evidence documenting that treatment reduces the provider-to-patient transmission risk.

The past decade has witnessed approaches to the therapy for chronic HCV infec-tion that have been increasingly encouraging. Success rates in therapy for chronic HCV infection approach 80%. In addition, published studies suggest that acute HCV infection can be successfully treated more than 95% of the time.[145–148] Because of these success rates, providers infected with HCV should certainly have a trial of treatment. Unlike HBV treatment, HCV therapy is often curative.

Strategies Designed to Reduce Risks by Restricting the Practices of Infected Providers

Current United States guidelines recommend that "health care providers who perform exposure-prone procedures and who do not have serologic evidence of immunity to HBV from vaccination or from previous infection should know their HBsAg status and, if that is positive, should also know their HBeAg status. If infected with HBV (and HBeAg positive) providers should not perform exposure-prone procedures unless they have sought counsel from an expert review panel and been advised under what circumstances, if any, they may continue to perform these procedures. Such circumstances would include notifying prospective patients of the health care worker's seropositivity before they undergo exposure-prone invasive procedures."[149] These guidelines were initially published in 1991 and have never been revised, despite the progress in the field since that time.

Several alternative sets of guidelines for managing HBV-infected providers have been published. United Kingdom guidelines restrict the practices of HBV-infected providers who are "e" antigen positive from performing exposure-prone invasive procedures. In these guidelines HBV-infected providers who are "e" antigen negative, but have HBV DNA levels greater than 10^3 genome-equivalents/mL, also are restricted from performing such procedures. HBV-infected providers who are "e" antigen negative and have HBV DNA levels of less than 10^3 are allowed to perform exposure-prone invasive procedures, as long as they are retested at least every 12 months to assure that their HBV viral burdens remain below 10^3.[150] Newer United Kingdom guidelines address the issue of antiviral therapy for HBV-infected providers and recommend that "e" antigen negative, HBV-infected health care providers whose pretreatment HBV DNA levels are between 10^3 and 10^5 genome-equivalents/mL may be permitted to perform exposure-prone invasive procedures if their viral burden on treatment falls to less than 10^3 genome equivalents/mL and if the provider remains on suppressive oral antiviral therapy.[151]

Another set of guidelines from a European consortium set slightly different thresholds.[152] These guidelines set the threshold for restriction for "e" antigen negative, HBV-infected providers at 10^4 genome-equivalents/mL.[152] Similar to the United States guidelines, the European guidelines also emphasize that providers who have been detected or implicated as having transmitted HBV should be restricted from performing exposure-prone procedures. The European guidelines recommend that HBV-infected providers who have received antiviral therapy and whose post-treatment DNA levels are less than 10^4 genome-equivalents/mL are permitted to perform exposure-prone procedures, so long as they are retested every 3 months to assure that their viral burden remains below 10^4.[152]

A set of recommendations published from the Netherlands set the restriction threshold for the conduct of exposure-prone invasive procedures at HBV DNA levels of less than 10^5.[153]

The Viral Hepatitis Prevention Board, a European consortium whose mission is to contribute to the control and prevention of viral hepatitis, recently identified several challenges that must be addressed to be able to standardize guidelines, including: (1) how to manage the variability in HBV DNA over time in HBV carriers; (2) how to address the limited data linking actual HBV viral burdens to the risk for health care–associated transmission; (3) the variation in reliability and reproducibility of molecular tests for HBV DNA, as well as the lack of standardization among these tests; and (4) how to manage providers on therapy because of the variability of the antiviral effects and the variable speed with which resistance develops.[154]

Although the 1991 US Public Health Service Guidelines made no recommendation regarding the management of individuals infected with hepatitis C, no United States guidelines have recommended practice restrictions for HCV-infected providers.[149] In contrast, the United Kingdom guidelines prohibit HCV-infected providers who have circulating HCV RNA from performing exposure-prone invasive procedures.[155] The United Kingdom guidelines also recommend that HCV-infected providers who receive antiviral treatment and become HCV RNA negative for 6 months can perform exposure-prone invasive procedures, but must be retested in 6 months to assure that the provider remains HCV RNA negative.[155] The European Consortium guidelines did not achieve consensus about HCV-infected providers, but concluded that HCV-infected providers not be restricted at this point in time.[152]

The existing evidence base is insufficient to permit the definitive selection of cutoffs for HBV or HCV viral burdens that are associated with risk for transmission. In one modeling study, the investigators suggested that a typical hollow-bore needlestick exposure to blood from an individual who had a viral burden of 10^4 genome-equivalents/mL would result in an exposure to less than one virion.[156] As indirect support for this concept, to date, every "e" antigen negative provider except one[157] who has been responsible for HBV provider-to-patient transmission has had a viral burden greater than 10^4.[152] The validity of the measurement of the one case that is the exception has been called into question, because the sample was drawn more than 3 months after the transmission.[153] Setting the HBV viral load cutoff at 10^3 results in practice restrictions for 58% of the HBV-infected providers in the United Kingdom and nearly 95% in the Netherlands.[154]

ADDITIONAL CHALLENGES

The concept of "exposure-prone" invasive procedures has been problematic since the issuance of the US Public Health Service Guidelines. Some authorities have suggested that providers, rather than procedures, might be exposure-prone, suggesting that technical expertise and experience may play a more substantive role in the risk for provider-to-patient exposure, rather than the procedures themselves. A panel of experts convened by the US CDC was unable to come to a consensus about which invasive procedures should be categorized as "exposure-prone." More recent guidelines and articles have suggested that exposure-prone procedures can be defined.[150,155,158,159] The United Kingdom guidelines characterized exposure-prone procedures[158] and, more recently, a multidisciplinary group created a table of procedures, divided into 3 categories: (1) procedures with *de minimis* risk of viral transmission; (2) procedures for which viral transmission is theoretically possible, but unlikely; and (3) procedures that are associated with a definite risk of viral transmission or that are directly characterized as exposure-prone procedures.[159]

Evaluating the cases of provider-to-patient transmission of these 2 viruses, the overwhelming majority of especially the more recent cases have been linked to major surgical procedures. For example, for the HCV cases (excluding those in which provider intravenous narcotics use was involved) 2 gynecologists, 3 cardiac or thoracic surgeons, an anesthesiologist, and an orthopedic surgeon were involved.

In the authors' view the creation and use of a so-called expert review panel has been an extremely useful aspect of the management of providers infected with bloodborne pathogens. The fact that very few instances of provider-to-patient transmission of either HBV or HCV have received publicity in the United States since the early part of this decade may provide indirect evidence for the utility of this approach. Such a panel could be centered at an institutional, municipal, county, state, or national level, consonant with local, state, and national laws. The panel, at a minimum, should include representation from hospital epidemiology, infectious diseases, the provider's specialty or subspecialty, occupational medicine (ie, the individual involved in monitoring the provider), hospital administration and, perhaps, legal and ethics representation as well. As each of these cases will have unique aspects, each should be considered independently. Important functions of the panel include: advising the health care provider, the occupational medicine physician, or the patient's primary physician about the provider's practice; advising the provider and her or his medical practitioner about the provider's capacity to conduct exposure-prone procedures; advising the provider about the appropriate use of infection control interventions; and considering the provider's performance at the time the provider's viral burden is measured.

New guidelines are sorely needed: guidelines that are based on firmer evidence, that synchronize the existing guidelines, and that are framed around the accumulating evidence that relates the risks for transmission to viral burden.

REFERENCES

1. Leibowitz S, Greenwald L, Cohen I, et al. Serum hepatitis in a blood bank worker. JAMA 1949;140:1331.
2. Dienstag JL, Ryan DM. Occupational exposure to hepatitis B virus in hospital personnel: infection or immunization. Am J Epidemiol 1982;115:26.
3. Hadler SC, Doto IL, Maynard JE, et al. Occupational risk of hepatitis B infection in hospital workers. Infect Control 1985;6:24.
4. Jovanovich JF, Saravolatz LD, Arking LM. The risk of hepatitis B among select employee groups in an urban hospital. JAMA 1983;250:1893.
5. Snydman DR, Muñoz A, Werner BG, et al. A multivariate analysis of risk factors for hepatitis B virus infection among hospital employees screened for vaccination. Am J Epidemiol 1984;120:684.
6. West DJ. The risk of hepatitis B infection among health professionals in the United States: a review. Am J Med Sci 1984;287:26.
7. Seeff LB, Wright EC, Zimmerman HJ, et al. Type B hepatitis after needlestick exposure: prevention with hepatitis B immune globulin: final report of the Veterans' Administration Cooperative Study. Ann Intern Med 1978;88:285.
8. Werner BJ, Grady GF. Accidental hepatitis-B-surface- antigen-positive inoculations: use of "e" antigen to estimate infectivity. Ann Intern Med 1982;97:367.
9. Transmission of hepatitis B to patients from four infected surgeons without hepatitis B e antigen. The Incident Investigation Teams and others. N Engl J Med 1997;336:178.
10. Cariani E, Zonaro A, Primi D, et al. Detection of HCV RNA and antibodies to HCV after needlestick injury. Lancet 1991;337:850.
11. Marranconi F, Mecenero V, Pellizzer GP, et al. HCV infection after accidental needlestick injury in health-care workers. Infection 1992;20:111.
12. Mizuno Y, Suzuki K, Mori M, et al. Study of needlestick accidents and hepatitis C virus infection in healthcare workers by molecular evolutionary analysis. J Hosp Infect 1997;35:149.
13. Nakano Y, Kiyosawa K, Sodeyama T, et al. Acute hepatitis C transmitted by needlestick accident despite short duration interferon treatment. J Gastroenterol Hepatol 1995;10:609.
14. Noguchi S, Sata M, Suzuki H, et al. Early therapy with interferon for acute hepatitis C acquired through a needlestick. Clin Infect Dis 1997;24:992.
15. Norder H, Bergstrom A, Uhnoo I, et al. Confirmation of nosocomial transmission of hepatitis C virus by phylogenetic analysis of the NS5-B region. J Clin Microbiol 1998;36:3066.
16. Ridzon R, Gallagher K, Ciesielski C, et al. Simultaneous transmission of human immunodeficiency virus and hepatitis C virus from a needle-stick injury. N Engl J Med 1997;336:919.
17. Schlipkoter U, Roggendorf M, Cholmakow K, et al. Transmission of hepatitis C virus (HCV) from a haemodialysis patient to a medical staff member. Scand J Infect Dis 1990;22:757.
18. Seeff LB. Hepatitis C from a needlestick injury. Ann Intern Med 1991;115:411.

19. Sulkowski MS, Ray SC, Thomas DL. Needlestick transmission of hepatitis C. JAMA 2002;287:2406.
20. Suzuki K, Mizokami M, Lau JY, et al. Confirmation of hepatitis C virus transmission through needlestick accidents by molecular evolutionary analysis. J Infect Dis 1994;170:1575.
21. Tsude K, Fujiyama S, Sato S, et al. Two cases of accidental transmission of hepatitis C to medical staff. Hepatogastroenterology 1992;39:73.
22. Vaqlia A, Nicolin R, Puro V, et al. Needlestick hepatitis C virus seroconversion in a surgeon. Lancet 1990;336:1315.
23. Seeff LB, Zimmerman HJ, Wright EC, et al. A randomized, double blind controlled trial of the efficacy of immune serum globulin for the prevention of post-transfusion hepatitis. Gastroenterology 1977;72:111.
24. Abacioglu YH, Bacaksiz F, Bahar IH, et al. Molecular evidence of nosocomial transmission of hepatitis C virus in a haemodialysis unit. Eur J Clin Microbiol Infect Dis 2000;19:182.
25. Allander T, Gruber A, Naghavi M, et al. Frequent patient-to-patient transmission of hepatitis C virus in a haematology ward. Lancet 1995;345:603.
26. Delarocque-Astagneau E, Baffoy N, Thiers V, et al. Outbreak of hepatitis C virus infection in a hemodialysis unit: potential transmission by the hemodialysis machine? Infect Control Hosp Epidemiol 2002;23:328.
27. Le Pogam S, Le Chapois D, Christen R, et al. Hepatitis C in a hemodialysis unit: molecular evidence for nosocomial transmission. J Clin Microbiol 1998;36:3040.
28. Wreghitt TG. Blood-borne virus infections in dialysis units—a review. Rev Med Virol 1999;9:101.
29. Tokars JI, Frank M, Alter MJ, et al. National surveillance of dialysis-associated diseases in the United States, 2000. Semin Dial 2002;15:162.
30. Henderson DK. Managing occupational risks for hepatitis C transmission in the healthcare setting. Clin Microbiol Rev 2003;16:546.
31. Bruguera M, Saiz JC, Franco S, et al. Outbreak of nosocomial hepatitis C virus infection resolved by genetic analysis of HCV RNA. J Clin Microbiol 2002;40:4363.
32. Dumpis U, Kovalova Z, Jansons J, et al. An outbreak of HBV and HCV infection in a paediatric oncology ward: epidemiological investigations and prevention of further spread. J Med Virol 2003;69:331.
33. Germain JM, Carbonne A, Thiers V, et al. Patient-to-patient transmission of hepatitis C virus through the use of multidose vials during general anesthesia. Infect Control Hosp Epidemiol 2005;26:789.
34. Katzenstein TL, Jorgensen LB, Permin H, et al. Nosocomial HIV-transmission in an outpatient clinic detected by epidemiological and phylogenetic analyses. AIDS 1999;13:1737.
35. Krause G, Trepka MJ, Whisenhunt RS, et al. Nosocomial transmission of hepatitis C virus associated with the use of multidose saline vials. Infect Control Hosp Epidemiol 2003;24:122.
36. Lagging LM, Aneman C, Nenonen N, et al. Nosocomial transmission of HCV in a cardiology ward during the window phase of infection: an epidemiological and molecular investigation. Scand J Infect Dis 2002;34:580.
37. Savey A, Simon F, Izopet J, et al. A large nosocomial outbreak of hepatitis C virus infections at a hemodialysis center. Infect Control Hosp Epidemiol 2005; 26:752.
38. Silini E, Locasciulli A, Santoleri L, et al. Hepatitis C virus infection in a hematology ward: evidence for nosocomial transmission and impact on hematologic disease outcome. Haematologica 2002;87:1200.

39. Centers for Disease Control. Patient exposures to HIV during nuclear medicine procedures. MMWR Morb Mortal Wkly Rep 1992;41:575.
40. Allander T, Medin C, Jacobson SH, et al. Transmission of hepatitis C virus by transfer of an infected individual to a new dialysis unit. Nephron 1996;73:110.
41. Alter MJ. Healthcare should not be a vehicle for transmission of hepatitis C virus. J Hepatol 2008;48:2.
42. Arai Y, Noda K, Enomoto N, et al. A prospective study of hepatitis C virus infection after needlestick accidents. Liver 1996;16:331.
43. Centers for Disease Control and Prevention. Acute hepatitis C virus infections attributed to unsafe injection practices at an endoscopy clinic—Nevada, 2007. MMWR Morb Mortal Wkly Rep 2008;57:513.
44. Desenclos JC, Bourdiol-Razes M, Rolin B, et al. Hepatitis C in a ward for cystic fibrosis and diabetic patients: possible transmission by spring-loaded finger-stick devices for self-monitoring of capillary blood glucose. Infect Control Hosp Epidemiol 2001;22:701.
45. Quer J, Esteban JI, Sanchez JM, et al. Nosocomial transmission of hepatitis C virus during contrast-enhanced computed tomography scanning. Eur J Gastroenterol Hepatol 2008;20:73.
46. Williams IT, Perz JF, Bell BP. Hepatitis C virus transmission from healthcare workers to patients in the United States. J Clin Virol 2006;36:S43.
47. Hutin YJ, Goldstein ST, Varma JK, et al. An outbreak of hospital-acquired hepatitis B virus infection among patients receiving chronic hemodialysis. Infect Control Hosp Epidemiol 1999;20:731.
48. Petrosillo N, Ippolito G, Solforosi L, et al. Molecular epidemiology of an outbreak of fulminant hepatitis B. J Clin Microbiol 2000;38:2975.
49. Quale JM, Landman D, Wallace B, et al. Deja vu: nosocomial hepatitis B virus transmission and fingerstick monitoring. Am J Med 1998;105:296.
50. Singh J, Bhatia R, Gandhi JC, et al. Outbreak of viral hepatitis B in a rural community in India linked to inadequately sterilized needles and syringes. Bull World Health Organ 1998;76:93.
51. Yerly S, Quadri R, Negro F, et al. Nosocomial outbreak of multiple bloodborne viral infections. J Infect Dis 2001;184:369.
52. Cerrai T, Michelassi S, Ierpi C, et al. Universal precautions and dedicated machines as cheap and effective measures to control HCV spread. EDTNA ERCA J 1998;24:43.
53. Djordjevic V, Stojanovic K, Stojanovic M, et al. Prevention of nosocomial transmission of hepatitis C infection in a hemodialysis unit. A prospective study. Int J Artif Organs 2000;23:181.
54. Fabrizi F, Martin P, Dixit V, et al. Acquisition of hepatitis C virus in hemodialysis patients: a prospective study by branched DNA signal amplification assay. Am J Kidney Dis 1998;31:647.
55. Fabrizi F, Martin P, Lunghi G, et al. Nosocomial transmission of hepatitis C virus infection in hemodialysis patients: clinical perspectives. Int J Artif Organs 2000;23:805.
56. Grethe S, Gemsa F, Monazahian M, et al. Molecular epidemiology of an outbreak of HCV in a hemodialysis unit: direct sequencing of HCV-HVR1 as an appropriate tool for phylogenetic analysis. J Med Virol 2000;60:152.
57. Halfon P, Roubicek C, Gerolami V, et al. Use of phylogenetic analysis of hepatitis C virus (HCV) hypervariable region 1 sequences to trace an outbreak of HCV in an autodialysis unit. J Clin Microbiol 2002;40:1541.

58. Irish DN, Blake C, Christophers J, et al. Identification of hepatitis C virus sero-conversion resulting from nosocomial transmission on a haemodialysis unit: implications for infection control and laboratory screening. J Med Virol 1999; 59:135.

59. Izopet J, Pasquier C, Sandres K, et al. Molecular evidence for nosocomial trans-mission of hepatitis C virus in a French hemodialysis unit. J Med Virol 1999;58: 139.

60. Katsoulidou A, Paraskevis D, Kalapothaki V, et al. Molecular epidemiology of a hepatitis C virus outbreak in a haemodialysis unit. Multicentre haemodialysis cohort study on viral hepatitis. Nephrol Dial Transplant 1999;14:1188.

61. McElborough D, Paul J, Hargreaves R, et al. Possible cross-infection with hepa-titis C virus of an unusual genotype on a haemodialysis unit. J Hosp Infect 2001; 47:335.

62. Petrosillo N, Gilli P, Serraino D, et al. Prevalence of infected patients and under-staffing have a role in hepatitis C virus transmission in dialysis. Am J Kidney Dis 2001;37:1004.

63. Sivapalasingam S, Malak SF, Sullivan JF, et al. High prevalence of hepatitis C infection among patients receiving hemodialysis at an urban dialysis center. Infect Control Hosp Epidemiol 2002;23:319.

64. Sullivan DG, Kim SS, Wilson JJ, et al. Investigating hepatitis C virus heteroge-neity in a high prevalence setting using heteroduplex tracking analysis. J Virol Methods 2001;96:5.

65. Taskapan H, Oymak O, Dogukan A, et al. Patient to patient transmission of hepatitis C virus in hemodialysis units. Clin Nephrol 2001;55:477.

66. Alfurayh O, Sabeel A, Al Ahdal MN, et al. Hand contamination with hepatitis C virus in staff looking after hepatitis C-positive hemodialysis patients. Am J Nephrol 2000;20:103.

67. Aucella F, Vigilante M, Valente GL, et al. Systematic monitor disinfection is effec-tive in limiting HCV spread in hemodialysis. Blood Purif 2000;18:110.

68. Tokars JI, Arduino MJ, Alter MJ. Infection control in hemodialysis units. Infect Dis Clin North Am 2001;15:797.

69. Bari A, Akhtar S, Rahbar MH, et al. Risk factors for hepatitis C virus infection in male adults in Rawalpindi-Islamabad, Pakistan. Trop Med Int Health 2001; 6:732.

70. Frank C, Mohamed MK, Strickland GT, et al. The role of parenteral antischisto-somal therapy in the spread of hepatitis C virus in Egypt. Lancet 2000;355:887.

71. Habib M, Mohamed MK, Abdel-Aziz F, et al. Hepatitis C virus infection in a community in the Nile Delta: risk factors for seropositivity. Hepatology 2001; 33:248.

72. Hutin YJ, Duclos P, Hogerzeil H, et al. Unsterile injections and emergence of human pathogens. Lancet 2002;359:2280.

73. Khan AJ, Luby SP, Fikree F, et al. Unsafe injections and the transmission of hepatitis B and C in a periurban community in Pakistan. Bull World Health Organ 2000;78:956.

74. Medhat A, Shehata M, Magder LS, et al. Hepatitis C in a community in Upper Egypt: risk factors for infection. Am J Trop Med Hyg 2002;66:633.

75. Mujeeb SA. Unsafe injections: a potential source of HCV spread in Pakistan. J Pak Med Assoc 2001;51:1.

76. Rao MR, Naficy AB, Darwish MA, et al. Further evidence for association of hepa-titis C infection with parenteral schistosomiasis treatment in Egypt. BMC Infect Dis 2002;2:29.

77. Petit JM, Bour JB, Aho LS, et al. HCV and diabetes mellitus: influence of noso-comial transmission with the use of a finger stick device. Am J Gastroenterol 1999;94:1709.
78. Lesourd F, Izopet J, Mervan C, et al. Transmissions of hepatitis C virus during the ancillary procedures for assisted conception. Hum Reprod 2000;15:1083.
79. Massari M, Petrosillo N, Ippolito G, et al. Transmission of hepatitis C virus in a gynecological surgery setting. J Clin Microbiol 2001;39:2860.
80. Public Health Laboratory Service. Transmission of hepatitis C virus from surgeon to patient prompts lookback. Commun Dis Rep CDR Wkly 1999;9:387.
81. Ross RS, Viazov S, Thormahlen M, et al. Risk of hepatitis C virus transmission from an infected gynecologist to patients: results of a 7-year retrospective inves-tigation. Arch Intern Med 2002;162:805.
82. Trasancos CC, Kainer MA, Desmond PV, et al. Investigation of potential iatro-genic transmission of hepatitis C in Victoria, Australia. Aust N Z J Public Health 2001;25:241.
83. Widell A, Christensson B, Wiebe T, et al. Epidemiologic and molecular investiga-tion of outbreaks of hepatitis C virus infection on a pediatric oncology service. Ann Intern Med 1999;130:130.
84. Schvarcz R, Johansson B, Nystrom B, et al. Nosocomial transmission of hepa-titis C virus. Infection 1997;25:74.
85. Bronowicki JP, Venard V, Botte C, et al. Patient-to-patient transmission of hepa-titis C virus during colonoscopy. N Engl J Med 1997;337:237.
86. Muscarella LF. Recommendations for preventing hepatitis C virus infection: analysis of a Brooklyn endoscopy clinic's outbreak. Infect Control Hosp Epidemiol 2001;22:669.
87. Bell D, Shapiro CN, Chamberland ME, et al. Preventing bloodborne pathogen transmission from health-care workers to patients: the CDC perspective. Surg Clin North Am 1995;75:1189.
88. American Academy of Orthopedic Surgeons Task Force on AIDS and Ortho-pedic Surgery. Recommendations for the prevention of human immunodefi-ciency virus (HIV) transmission in the practice of orthopedic surgery 1989. Park Ridge (IL): American Academy of Orthopedic Surgeons.
89. Harpaz R, Von Seidlein L, Averhoff FM, et al. Transmission of hepatitis B virus to multiple patients from a surgeon without evidence of inadequate infection control. N Engl J Med 1996;334:549.
90. Johnston B, Langille D, LeBlanc J, et al. Transmission of hepatitis B related to orthopedic surgery [abstract]. Infect Control Hosp Epidemiol 1994;15:352.
91. Bosch X. Hepatitis C outbreak astounds Spain. Lancet 1998;351:1415.
92. Brown P. Surgeon infects patient with hepatitis C. BMJ 1999;319:1219.
93. Cody SH, Nainan OV, Garfein RS, et al. Hepatitis C virus transmission from an anesthesiologist to a patient. Arch Intern Med 2002;162:345.
94. Duckworth GJ, Heptonstall J, Aitken C. Transmission of hepatitis C virus from a surgeon to a patient. The incident control team. Commun Dis Public Health 1999;2:188.
95. Esteban JI, Gomez J, Martell M, et al. Transmission of hepatitis C virus by a cardiac surgeon. N Engl J Med 1996;334:555.
96. Mawdsley J, Teo CG, Kyi M, et al. Anesthetist to patient transmission of hepatitis C virus associated with non exposure-prone procedures. J Med Virol 2005;75:399.
97. Public Health Laboratory Service. Hepatitis C lookback exercise. Commun Dis Rep CDR Wkly 2000;10:203.

98. Public Health Laboratory Service. Hepatitis C lookback in two trusts in the south of England, vol. 12 (34). London (UK): Public Health Laboratory Service, 2002.

99. Public Health Laboratory Service. Hepatitis C transmission from health care worker to patient. Commun Dis Rep CDR Wkly 1995;5:121.

100. Public Health Laboratory Service. Two hepatitis C lookback exercises—national and in London. Commun Dis Rep CDR Wkly 2000;10:125.

101. Ross RS, Viazov S, Roggendorf M. Phylogenetic analysis indicates transmission of hepatitis C virus from an infected orthopedic surgeon to a patient. J Med Virol 2002;66:461.

102. Shemer-Avni Y, Cohen M, Keren-Naus A, et al. Iatrogenic transmission of hepatitis C virus (HCV) by an anesthesiologist: comparative molecular analysis of the HCV-E1 and HCV-E2 hypervariable regions. Clin Infect Dis 2007;45:e32.

103. Williams IT, Perz JF, Bell BP. Viral hepatitis transmission in ambulatory health care settings. Clin Infect Dis 2004;38:1592.

104. Centers for Disease Control. Update: universal precautions for prevention of transmission of human immunodeficiency virus, hepatitis B virus, and other bloodborne pathogens in health-care settings. MMWR Morb Mortal Wkly Rep 1988;37:377.

105. Kovavisarach E, Jaravechson S. Comparison of perforation between single and double-gloving in perineorrhaphy after vaginal delivery: a randomized controlled trial. Aust N Z J Obstet Gynaecol 1998;38:58.

106. Kovavisarach E, Seedadee C. Randomised controlled trial of glove perforation in single and double-gloving methods in gynaecologic surgery. Aust N Z J Obstet Gynaecol 2002;42:519.

107. Kovavisarach E, Vanitchanon P. Perforation in single- and double-gloving methods for cesarean section. Int J Gynaecol Obstet 1999;67:157.

108. Kristensen MS, Wernberg NM, Anker ME. Healthcare workers' risk of contact with body fluids in a hospital: the effect of complying with the universal precautions policy. Infect Control Hosp Epidemiol 1992;13:719.

109. Ross RS, Viazov S, Gross T, et al. Transmission of hepatitis C virus from a patient to an anesthesiology assistant to five patients. N Engl J Med 2000;343:1851.

110. Bosch X. Newspaper apportions blame in Spanish hepatitis C scandal. Lancet 2000;355:818.

111. Centers for Disease Control. Recommendations for prevention of HIV transmission in health-care settings. MMWR Morb Mortal Wkly Rep 1987;36(Suppl 2):1S.

112. Centers for Disease Control. Recommendations for protection against viral hepatitis. MMWR Morb Mortal Wkly Rep 1985;34:313.

113. Garner JS. Guideline for isolation precautions in hospitals. The Hospital Infection Control Practices Advisory Committee. Infect Control Hosp Epidemiol 1996;17:53.

114. Beekmann SE, Vlahov D, Koziol DE, et al. Temporal association between implementation of universal precautions and a sustained, progressive decrease in percutaneous exposures to blood. Clin Infect Dis 1994;18:562.

115. Haiduven DJ, DeMaio TM, Stevens DA. A five-year study of needlestick injuries: significant reduction associated with communication, education, and convenient placement of sharps containers. Infect Control Hosp Epidemiol 1992;13:265.

116. Wong ES, Stotka JL, Mayhall CG, et al. Cost-efficacy of hospital infection control before and after the implementation of universal precautions. Abstract 786. In: 29th Interscience Conference on antimicrobial agents and chemotherapy. Houston, Texas, September 17–20, 1989. p. 233.

117. Akduman D, Kim LE, Parks RL, et al. Use of personal protective equipment and operating room behaviors in four surgical subspecialties: personal protective equipment and behaviors in surgery. Infect Control Hosp Epidemiol 1999;20:110.

118. Davis JM, Demling RH, Lewis FR, et al. The Surgical Infection Society's policy on human immunodeficiency virus and hepatitis B and C infection. The Ad Hoc Committee on acquired immunodeficiency syndrome and hepatitis. Arch Surg 1992;127:218.

119. Hester RA, Nelson CL, Harrison S. Control of contamination of the operative team in total joint arthroplasty. J Arthroplasty 1992;7:267.

120. Lewis FR Jr, Short LJ, Howard RJ, et al. Epidemiology of injuries by needles and other sharp instruments. Minimizing sharp injuries in gynecologic and obstetric operations. Surg Clin North Am 1995;75:1105.

121. Loudon MA, Stonebridge PA. Minimizing the risk of penetrating injury to surgical staff in the operating theatre: towards sharp-free surgery. J R Coll Surg Edinb 1998;43:6.

122. Tobias AM, Chang B. Pulsed irrigation of extremity wounds: a simple technique for splashback reduction. Ann Plast Surg 2002;48:443.

123. Aarnio P, Laine T. Glove perforation rate in vascular surgery—a comparison between single and double gloving. Vasa 2001;30:122.

124. Avery CM, Taylor J, Johnson PA. Double gloving and a system for identifying glove perforations in maxillofacial trauma surgery. Br J Oral Maxillofac Surg 1999;37:316.

125. Chapman S, Duff P. Frequency of glove perforations and subsequent blood contact in association with selected obstetric surgical procedures. Am J Obstet Gynecol 1993;168:1354.

126. Cohen MS, Do JT, Tahery DP, et al. Efficacy of double gloving as a protection against blood exposure in dermatologic surgery. J Dermatol Surg Oncol 1992;18:873.

127. Gerberding JL, Littell C, Tarkington A, et al. Risk of exposure of surgical personnel to patients' blood during surgery at San Francisco General Hospital. N Engl J Med 1990;322:1788.

128. Hollaus PH, Lax F, Janakiev D, et al. Glove perforation rate in open lung surgery. Eur J Cardiothorac Surg 1999;15:461.

129. Laine T, Aarnio P. How often does glove perforation occur in surgery? Comparison between single gloves and a double-gloving system. Am J Surg 2001;181:564.

130. Naver LP, Gottrup F. Incidence of glove perforations in gastrointestinal surgery and the protective effect of double gloves: a prospective, randomised controlled study. Eur J Surg 2000;166:293.

131. Gerberding JL, Quebbeman EJ, Rhodes RS. Hand protection. Surg Clin North Am 1995;75:1133.

132. Leslie LF, Woods JA, Thacker JG, et al. Needle puncture resistance of surgical gloves, finger guards, and glove liners. J Biomed Mater Res 1996;33:41.

133. Salkin JA, Stuchin SA, Kummer FJ, et al. The effectiveness of cut-proof glove liners: cut and puncture resistance, dexterity, and sensibility. Orthopedics 1995;18:1067.

134. Woods JA, Leslie LF, Drake DB, et al. Effect of puncture resistant surgical gloves, finger guards, and glove liners on cutaneous sensibility and surgical psychomotor skills. J Biomed Mater Res 1996;33:47.

135. Gerberding JL. Procedure-specific infection control for preventing intraoperative blood exposures. Am J Infect Control 1993;21:364.

136. Henderson DK. The AIDS/Tuberculosis Subcommittee of the Society for Health-care Epidemiology of America: management of healthcare workers infected with hepatitis B virus, hepatitis C virus, human immunodeficiency virus, or other bloodborne pathogens. AIDS/TB Committee of the Society for Healthcare Epidemiology of America. Infect Control Hosp Epidemiol 1997;18:349.

137. Centers for Disease Control and Prevention. Evaluation of blunt suture needles in preventing percutaneous injuries among health-care workers during gyneco-logic surgical procedures—New York City, March 1993-June 1994. MMWR Morb Mortal Wkly Rep 1997;46:25.

138. Hartley JE, Ahmed S, Milkins R, et al. Randomized trial of blunt-tipped versus cutting needles to reduce glove puncture during mass closure of the abdomen. Br J Surg 1996;83:1156.

139. Miller SS, Sabharwal A. Subcuticular skin closure using a 'blunt' needle. Ann R Coll Surg Engl 1994;76:281.

140. Mingoli A, Sapienza P, Sgarzini G, et al. Influence of blunt needles on surgical glove perforation and safety for the surgeon. Am J Surg 1996;172:512.

141. Montz FJ, Fowler JM, Farias-Eisner R, et al. Blunt needles in fascial closure. Surg Gynecol Obstet 1991;173:147.

142. Wright KU, Moran CG, Briggs PJ. Glove perforation during hip arthroplasty. A randomised prospective study of a new taperpoint needle. J Bone Joint Surg Br 1993;75:918.

143. Department of Labor OSHA. Occupational exposure to bloodborne pathogens; final rule. Fed Regist 1991;56:64175.

144. Hoofnagle JH, Doo E, Liang TJ, et al. Management of hepatitis B: summary of a clinical research workshop. Hepatology 2007;45:1056.

145. Alberti A, Boccato S, Vario A, et al. Therapy of acute hepatitis C. Hepatology 2002;36:S195.

146. Fabris P. Acute hepatitis C: epidemiology, pathogenesis and therapy. Curr Pharm Des 2008;14:1644.

147. Jaeckel E, Cornberg M, Wedemeyer H, et al. Treatment of acute hepatitis C with interferon alfa-2b. N Engl J Med 2001;345:1452.

148. Wiegand J, Deterding K, Cornberg M, et al. Treatment of acute hepatitis C: the success of monotherapy with (pegylated) interferon alpha. J Antimicrob Chemother 2008;62:860.

149. Centers for Disease Control. Recommendations for preventing transmission of human immunodeficiency virus and hepatitis B virus to patients during expo-sure-prone invasive procedures. MMWR Morb Mortal Wkly Rep 1991;40:1.

150. Department of Health (UK). Hepatitis B infected health care workers: guidance on implementation of health service circular 2000/020. Health UK Department of Health. London, 2000, vol. 2009.

151. Department of Health (UK). Hepatitis B infected healthcare workers and antiviral therapy. Health UK Department of Health. London, 2007, vol. 2009

152. Gunson RN, Shouval D, Roggendorf M, et al. Hepatitis B virus (HBV) and hepa-titis C virus (HCV) infections in health care workers (HCWs): guidelines for prevention of transmission of HBV and HCV from HCW to patients. J Clin Virol 2003;27:213.

153. Buster EH, van der Eijk AA, Schalm SW. Doctor to patient transmission of hepa-titis B virus: implications of HBV DNA levels and potential new solutions. Antiviral Res 2003;60:79.

154. FitzSimons D, Francois G, De Carli G, et al. Hepatitis B virus, hepatitis C virus and other blood-borne infections in healthcare workers: guidelines for

prevention and management in industrialised countries. Occup Environ Med 2008;65:446.

155. Department of Health (UK). Hepatitis C infected health care workers. Health UK Department of Health. Health Service Circular. London, 2002, vol. 2009.

156. Bennett NT, Howard RJ. Quantity of blood inoculated in a needlestick injury from suture needles. J Am Coll Surg 1994;178:107.

157. Corden S, Ballard AL, Ijaz S, et al. HBV DNA levels and transmission of hepatitis B by health care workers. J Clin Virol 2003;27:52.

158. Department of Health (UK). HIV infected health care workers: guidance on management and patient notification. Health UK Department of Health. Health Service Circular. London, 2005, vol. 2009.

159. Reitsma AM, Closen ML, Cunningham M, et al. Infected physicians and invasive procedures: safe practice management. Clin Infect Dis 2005;40:1665.

US Outbreak Investigations Highlight the Need for Safe Injection Practices and Basic Infection Control

Joseph F. Perz, DrPH, MA[a],*, Nicola D. Thompson, PhD, MS[b], Melissa K. Schaefer, MD[a,c], Priti R. Patel, MD, MPH[a]

KEYWORDS

- Hepatitis B virus • Hepatitis C virus • Injections
- Infection control • Outbreak

Preventing the spread of bloodborne pathogens, particularly hepatitis B virus (HBV), hepatitis C virus (HCV), and human immunodeficiency virus (HIV), represents a basic expectation anywhere health care is provided. This is true both in terms of patient and provider protections. Health care should provide no avenue for the transmission of these potentially life-threatening infections; yet, unsafe medical practices continue to contribute to much of the worldwide disease burden that is associated with HBV and HCV.[1,2] Even in wealthy countries, such as the United States, the challenge of consistently providing safe care is not always met, as evidenced by increasing reports of outbreaks that have been associated with unsafe injection practices and related breakdowns in basic infection control.[3,4]

Current understanding of viral hepatitis transmission in United States health care settings indicates progress over the past several decades with respect to the risks from transfusions or blood products.[5,6] Likewise, risks to health care providers from

The findings and conclusions of this article are those of the authors and do not necessarily represent the official position of the Centers for Disease Control and Prevention.

[a] Division of Healthcare Quality Promotion, Prevention and Response Branch, Centers for Disease Control and Prevention, 1600 Clifton Road, MS A-31, Atlanta, GA 30333, USA

[b] Division of Viral Hepatitis, Epidemiology and Surveillance Branch, Centers for Disease Control and Prevention, 1600 Clifton Road, MS G-37, Atlanta, GA 30333, USA

[c] Epidemic Intelligence Service, Office of Workforce and Career Development, Centers for Disease Control and Prevention, 1600 Clifton Road, MS E-92, Atlanta, GA 30333, USA

* Corresponding author.

E-mail address: jperz@cdc.gov (J.F. Perz).

sharps injuries and other blood and body fluid exposures have been reduced as a consequence of widespread hepatitis B vaccination and the adoption of safer work practices.[3] Increasing recognition of outbreaks involving patient-to-patient spread of HBV and HCV infections, however, has uncovered a disturbing trend. This article highlights the importance of basic infection control and the need for increased awareness of safe injection practices.

OUTBREAKS: RECENT UNITED STATES EXPERIENCE

The detection of outbreaks of health care–associated viral hepatitis is haphazard; many barriers exist that hinder effective public health surveillance and investigation.[3,4] Most new infections are asymptomatic and there is a low index of suspicion for health care–associated bloodborne virus transmission among patients and providers. Outbreaks and sporadic transmission events are likely underrecognized.[4,7,8] Nonetheless, a recent review of United States viral hepatitis outbreak experience revealed 33 outbreaks that occurred in nonhospital settings, such as outpatient clinics (N = 12); dialysis centers (N = 6); and long-term care facilities (N = 15).[4] These outbreaks resulted in 448 recognized cases of HBV or HCV infection during 1998 to 2008.

Increasingly, these events have resulted in large public health notifications and facility closures.[4] Between 2007 and 2009, outpatient clinics were identified as the sites of at least four outbreaks of HBV or HCV infections that resulted from unsafe practices, such as improper use of syringes, needles, and medication vials.[4,9–11] In these incidents, many tens of thousands of patients were needlessly placed at risk for infection because of unsafe medical practices and were sent letters advising them to undergo testing for HBV, HCV, and HIV. For example, over 40,000 patients were impacted by an outbreak of HCV infections that occurred in an endoscopy clinic in Nevada.[9] Most recently, a chemotherapy clinic has become the epicenter of a hepatitis B outbreak investigation; approximately 6000 cancer patients who received treatment at this clinic have been contacted and recommended to undergo testing.[11] In turn, the media, legislators, and other officials have noted a public health crisis in affected communities where confidence in the health care system, including routine preventive services, has been undermined.

The outbreaks with the most widespread impact have occurred in outpatient settings, where attention to infection control is lacking relative to inpatient settings.[3,12,13] In these settings, transmission of HBV and HCV has been attributed to syringe reuse or other infection control lapses that resulted in contamination of injectable medications or flush solutions.[3,4,7,14] The delivery of anesthesia was a common factor in approximately half of these outbreaks.[4] Physicians and other health care providers should be aware of the potential consequences of unsafe injection practices. Besides compromising patient safety, unsafe care may also put providers themselves at risk of licensing board actions or malpractice suits (**Box 1**).

SYRINGE REUSE

The risks associated with syringe reuse and, more generally, the risks associated with improperly handled injectable medications, seem to be underappreciated (**Box 2**).[14,15] Essentially, any form of syringe reuse is a dangerous practice. A misperception that may underlie some of the risky behaviors is the mistaken belief that contamination is limited to the needle device when a syringe and needle are used as unit. Instead, as was demonstrated by decades old experimental studies, contamination does extend to the syringe when injections are administered by the intramuscular, intradermal, intravenous (IV), or other routes.[16–24] Additional potential for

---

Box 1
Injection safety information for providers

Several recent investigations undertaken by state and local health departments and the Centers for Disease Control and Prevention have identified improper use of syringes, needles, and medication vials during routine health care procedures, such as administering injections. These practices have resulted in one or more of the following:

- Transmission of bloodborne viruses, including hepatitis C virus, to patients

- Notification of thousands of patients of possible exposure to bloodborne pathogens and recommendation that they be tested for HCV, HBV, and HIV

- Referral of providers to licensing boards for disciplinary action

- Malpractice suits filed by patients

These unfortunate events serve as a reminder of the serious consequences of failure to maintain strict adherence to safe injection practices during patient care. Injection safety and other basic infection control practices are central to patient safety. All health care providers are urged to carefully review their infection control practices and the practices of all staff under their supervision. In particular, providers should ensure that staff:

- Never administer medications from the same syringe to more than one patient, even if the needle is changed

- Do not enter a vial with a used syringe or needle

HCV, HBV, and HIV can be spread from patient to patient when these simple precautions are not followed. Additional protection is offered when medication vials can be dedicated to a single patient. It is important that:

- Medications packaged as single-use vials never be used for more than one patient

- Medications packaged as multiuse vials be assigned to a single patient whenever possible

- Bags or bottles of intravenous solution not be used as a common source of supply for more than one patient

- Absolute adherence to proper infection control practices be maintained during the preparation and administration of injected medications

Data from CDC, March 2008. Available at: http://www.cdc.gov/ncidod/dhqp/ps_providerInfo.html.

---

syringe contamination results from the negative pressure that occurs if a contaminated needle is removed from the syringe. In the case of IV administration, the risk for syringe contamination is not eliminated by intervening lengths of IV tubing or the presence of heparin locks or valves.[21] Use of a contaminated needle or syringe to withdraw medication from a vial can result in transfer of contaminants to the vial, as shown in **Fig. 1**.[22]

Overt Reuse of Syringes

Reuse of syringes is a primary example of an unsafe injection practice that has resulted in HBV and HCV transmission. Overt syringe reuse involves reuse of a single syringe to administer parenteral medication or flush solutions to more than one patient. The danger of this practice was made clear in an Oklahoma outbreak that was investigated in 2002.[7,25] Here, an anesthetist in a pain remediation clinic routinely prepared a single needle and syringe at the beginning of each clinic session for each of three medications: midazolam, fentanyl, and propofol. These three needles and

---

Box 2
Injection safety for providers: frequently asked questions

What is injection safety? Injection safety, or safe injection practices, is a set of measures taken to perform injections in an optimally safe manner for patients, health care personnel, and others. A safe injection does not harm the recipient, does not expose the provider to any avoidable risks, and does not result in waste that is dangerous for the community. Injection safety includes practices intended to prevent transmission of infectious diseases between one patient and another, or between a patient and health care provider, and also to prevent harm, such as needlestick injuries.

What is aseptic technique? In this context, aseptic technique refers to the manner of handling medications and injection equipment to prevent microbial contamination. Aseptic technique applies to the handling, preparation, and storage of medications. It also applies to the handling of all supplies used for injections and infusions, including syringes, needles, and IV tubing.

What are some of the incorrect practices that have resulted in transmission of pathogens? Practices that have resulted in transmission of HCV or HBV include the following:

- Using the same syringe to administer medication to more than one patient, even if the needle was changed
- Using the same medication vial for more than one patient, and accessing the vial with a syringe that has already been used to administer medication to a patient
- Using a common bag of saline or other IV fluid for more than one patient, and accessing the bag with a syringe that has already been used to flush a patient's catheter

For what types of procedures have these incorrect practices been identified? Unsafe injection practices that put patients at risk for HCV, HBV, and other infections have been identified during various types of procedures. Examples include the following:

- Administration of anesthetics for outpatient surgical, diagnostic, and pain management procedures
- Administration of other IV medications for chemotherapy, cosmetic procedures, and alternative medicine therapies
- Use of saline to flush IV lines and catheters
- Administration of intramuscular vaccines

The involved medications were in single-use vials, multidose vials, and bags. What they had in common was the vials or bags were used for more than one patient and were entered with a syringe that had already been used for a patient; or the syringe itself was used for more than one patient.

Where should I draw up medications? Medications should be drawn up in a designated clean medication area that is not adjacent to areas where potentially contaminated items are placed. Examples of contaminated items that should not be placed in or near the medication preparation area include used equipment, such as syringes, needles, IV tubing, blood collection tubes, needle holders (eg, Vacutainer holder), or other soiled equipment or materials that have been used in a procedure. In general, any item that could have come in contact with blood or body fluids should not be in the medication preparation area.

Data from CDC, March 2008. Available at: http://www.cdc.gov/ncidod/dhqp/ps_providerInfo.html.

---

syringes were used to administer these medications sequentially to all patients treated in an individual clinic session, through a peripheral IV catheter. Over 100 HBV and HCV infections were transmitted in this manner over a 3-year period.[25]

A number of recent incidents involving overt syringe reuse have resulted in patient notifications, in the absence of clear evidence of transmitted infections, because of the

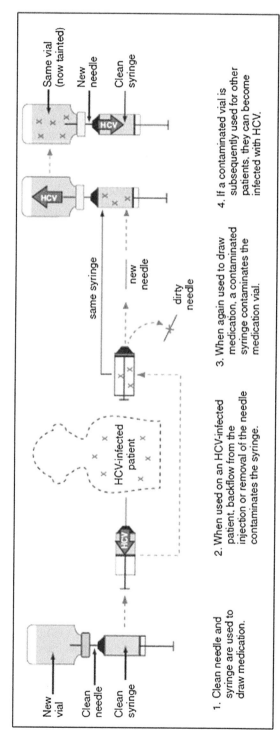

Fig. 1. Illustration of how indirect syringe reuse can lead to HCV contamination of a shared medication vial. (*Data from* Centers for Disease Control and Prevention (CDC). Acute hepatitis C virus infections attributed to unsafe injection practices at an endoscopy clinic—Nevada, 2007. MMWR Morbid Mortal Weekly Rep 2008;57:513–7.)

inherent risks. One such incident involved influenza vaccine that was drawn from a multidose vial into a 3-mL syringe that was then used to administer 0.5-mL unit doses to multiple patients, with the needle changed between patients.[26] Another incident involved a Michigan dermatologist who was suspected of reusing syringes; this resulted in approximately 13,500 patient notifications.[27] Several recent incidents involved the reuse of insulin pens, which are single patient-use items, for multiple patients.[28] Providers reported that they believed that changing the needles on the device was sufficient to prevent the transmission of infection. Several thousand patients were notified in these incidents. The Food and Drug Administration issued an alert reminding providers that insulin pens and cartridges must not be shared because of the risk of transmitting bloodborne pathogens and that the same risk may exist with shared use of any injection device.[29,30]

Contamination of Shared Medications by Reused Syringes

The reuse of syringes to withdraw medication or solutions has also repeatedly been shown to result in HBV and HCV transmission. This type of error does not typically involve overt reuse of the syringe for multiple patients as described previously. Instead, the syringe is reused to draw up additional medication for a single patient, administered, and then discarded. Because this action can contaminate the vial or bag containing the medication or solution, subsequent patients can be exposed to infectious virus or other microbes if that vial or bag is reused (see **Box 1**). Numerous outbreaks have been associated with this practice. For example, in a Nevada endoscopy center outbreak investigated in 2008, it was discovered that two nurse anesthetists routinely reused syringes, after changing needles, to obtain additional doses of propofol for individual patients who required additional sedation.[9] Although the syringe was discarded at the end of the procedure, any remaining medication in the single-dose propofol vial was used for subsequent patients. Patient-to-patient transmission of HCV on two separate days was documented using epidemiologic data and supported with viral sequencing results. Over 40,000 patients who had undergone procedures at this facility were potentially exposed to this long-standing practice and placed at risk of bloodborne pathogen transmission.[9] In another example, 99 patients treated at a hematology-oncology clinic in Nebraska were infected with HCV after a nurse reused syringes, after drawing blood from central venous catheters, to withdraw saline solution from 500-mL bags for flush procedures.[7,31,32] Each bag of saline solution was routinely used as a common source of flush for 25 to 50 patients.[31]

Transmission potential is magnified when facilities use vials or bags of medication and infusates that contain quantities in excess of those needed for routine single-patient use. Although these medications are often labeled as single-use (ie, single-dose), the large volume in the container may lead to the perception that they are suitable for multipatient use.[33] Large-volume single-dose or multidose medications are particularly risky because syringe reuse or other breaches in aseptic technique may result in a large reservoir of contaminated material that serves to perpetuate transmission to multiple patients. To reduce costs, some providers have pooled leftover contents from multiple vials to obtain a sufficient dose, risking serial contamination of additional vials and putting further patients at risk.[34,35] It is important that single-dose containers only be used once for a single procedure on a single patient (**Box 3**).[36] Additionally, the Centers for Disease Control and Prevention (CDC) recommends limiting use of multidose vials of medication to single patients to offer an extra barrier of protection against unrecognized syringe reuse or other means of contamination.

> **Box 3**
> **Injection safety recommendations**
>
> - Never administer medications from the same syringe to more than one patient, even if the needle is changed.
> - Consider a syringe or needle contaminated after it has been used to enter or connect to a patients' intravenous catheter, infusion bag or administration set.
> - Do not enter a vial with a used syringe or needle.
> - Never use medications packaged as single-use vials for more than one patient.
> - Assign medications packaged as multi-use vials to a single patient whenever possible.
> - Do not use bags or bottles of intravenous solution as a common source of supply for more than one patient.
> - Follow proper infection-control practices during the preparation and administration of injected medications.
>
> *Adapted from* Centers for Disease Control and Prevention. Guideline for isolation precautions: preventing transmission of infectious agents in healthcare settings 2007. Atlanta (GA): US Department of Health and Human Services, CDC; 2007. Available at: http://www.cdc.gov/ncidod/dhqp/gl_isolation.html.

CONTAMINATION OF EQUIPMENT, SUPPLIES, AND THE ENVIRONMENT

Equipment, supplies, and the environment can become contaminated and facilitate HBV and HCV transmission.[3,4] For example, in an outbreak that occurred in a private medical practice, 38 patients acquired HBV infection from injections that typically combined vitamins and steroids prepared using multidose vials that were stored in a workspace where used needles and syringes were dismantled and discarded.[37] Injections should be prepared in a clean environment that is not adjacent to areas where potentially contaminated items are placed (see **Box 2**).[36] If multidose vials are used to prepare IV medications for multiple patients, these should be restricted to a centralized medication area.[36] Unless these multidose vials are dedicated to a single patient, they should not enter the patient treatment or procedure area. In hemodialysis settings where blood contamination can occur frequently in patient care areas, neither multidose nor single-dose medications should be handled at the patient treatment station.[35,38] Standard Precautions also indicate that vials should be stored in accordance with manufacturer's recommendations (eg, held at room temperature or under refrigeration) and that vials should be discarded whenever sterility has been compromised or is in doubt.[36] Providers should be aware that the bacteriostatic agents used in multidose vials are not effective against viruses, such as HCV and HBV.

Bloodborne pathogen transmission also results from improper use and handling of patient equipment in the context of blood glucose monitoring.[4,28,39–44] Transmission has occurred when (1) equipment designed for use by a single person (eg, spring-loaded fingerstick devices; blood glucose meters) was inappropriately used for multiple patients; (2) equipment used for multiple patients (eg, blood glucose meters) was not cleaned and disinfected between each use; and (3) staff failed to wear gloves, change gloves, or perform hand hygiene for fingerstick procedures. Although transmission of this type has most clearly been recognized in long-term care facilities, conditions that could facilitate sporadic transmission by blood glucose monitoring and related diabetes care may be present in a wide array of settings, including hospitals.[28,45] In addition, although bloodborne pathogen transmission has not been reported in association with prothrombin time and International Normalized Ratio (INR) point-of-care testing devices, the increased use of these devices deserves attention. Their similarity to blood glucose monitoring equipment suggests a need for appropriate procedures to prevent transmission in physicians' offices, anticoagulation clinics, long-term care, and other settings where these devices are used.

This points to another misperception that likely contributes to health care–associated bloodborne virus transmission: cleaning of equipment and shared devices is only necessary when blood or other contamination is visible. This is not true. For example, one study, which used an assay to detect occult blood, found that 30% of blood glucose meters in routine use in hospitals were contaminated with blood.[46] Further, HBV and HCV have been shown to remain infectious in the environment in dry blood for up to a week and 16 hours, respectively; either virus may be present in the absence of visible blood in sufficient quantities to cause infection.[3,47,48] The CDC recommends that blood glucose meters should only be used for multiple patients if they are cleaned and disinfected after every use, because these devices frequently become contaminated with blood.[43] According to Standard Precautions, facilities should establish policies and procedures for containing, transporting, and handling all patient-care equipment, instruments, and devices that may be contaminated with blood or body fluids.[36] Additional recommendations that specifically address safe blood glucose monitoring and diabetes care are available and emphasize the importance of single-use autodisabling lancets, avoidance of shared blood glucose meters, appropriate hand hygiene, and safe injection practices for insulin delivery.[43]

Indirect contact transmission, such as that observed in the hemodialysis environment, can occur when proper attention is not given to the cleaning and disinfection of equipment, supplies, and the hands of health care personnel.[4,36,38,49–52] Patients receiving long-term hemodialysis, whose care involves repeated and prolonged vascular access in an environment that is shared with other patients, have historically been at high risk for acquiring bloodborne infection. Infection control recommendations for the hemodialysis setting have been established and were incorporated into recently revised Centers for Medicare and Medicaid Services (CMS) Conditions for Coverage for end-stage renal disease facilities.[25,38] The new requirements underscore the importance of proper medication handling and environmental decontamination and establish a framework for enforcing appropriate practices in this setting.

Care of the environment and adherence to Standard Precautions is important wherever health care is delivered.[36] Certain health care settings may be associated with higher risks for transmission, however, not only by virtue of the procedures performed, but also the underlying prevalence among the patient population. For example, a prospective study of patients treated in 308 representative dialysis facilities in the United States and several other developed nations found that higher facility HCV prevalence was independently predictive of incident HCV infections.[53] This finding highlights that opportunities for potential transmission increase as the prevalence of HCV-infected patients in a facility grows. Hepatology treatment centers may also have a high prevalence of HCV-infected patients and multiple opportunities for cross-contamination.[54,55] As such, these facilities should take special care to ensure complete adherence to safe injection practices, environmental cleaning, appropriate care of invasive equipment, and other recommended precautions.[36,38,55–57]

Endoscope reprocessing is another area that warrants specific attention. Failures to adhere to endoscope reprocessing guidelines have been associated with numerous outbreaks of bacterial infections.[58,59] Patient notifications and concerns over bloodborne pathogen transmission have also resulted from these types of lapses.[60] There has been little convincing evidence that endoscopes alone have served as the source of HBV or HCV transmission; unsafe injection practices including syringe reuse may have been overlooked in several incidents.[14,58,60,61] The risk of bloodborne pathogen transmission from endoscopes that have been appropriately cleaned but not undergone high-level disinfection is likely very small.[58,60–62] Nonetheless, reprocessing failures can pose a number of other infectious disease risks and resulting notifications can have widespread adverse impacts on patients and their family members. Recent examples have involved US Department of Veterans Affairs medical facilities in which over 10,000 patients were notified and offered bloodborne pathogen testing because they were exposed to improperly reprocessed endoscopy equipment.[63] Health care providers and institutions must ensure that their staff are appropriately trained in and adhere to recommended endoscope reprocessing procedures as part of their basic infection control and patient safety program.[57–59,64]

THE CLINICIAN'S ROLE IN IDENTIFYING HEALTH CARE–ASSOCIATED INFECTIONS

Clinicians can play a key role in helping to recognize and contain health care–associated viral hepatitis infections by reporting potential clusters or incident cases. The outbreaks that are investigated by health departments and the CDC likely underrepresent the true burden of health care–associated HCV and HBV infections in the United States.[4] Although traditional risk factors, such as high-risk sexual behaviors and injection-drug use, still contribute to the current epidemiology of acute HBV and HCV infections, approximately 50% of persons interviewed do not report behavioral risks as part of routine case-investigations for acute hepatitis B or C.[65] Unacknowledged behavioral risk factors likely explain a portion of the cases without identified risks or exposures, but unrecognized medical transmission might also account for many of these cases.[4] This should serve as a reminder to physicians diagnosing patients with acute viral hepatitis to report these cases and carefully consider the role of health care exposures, especially among older adult populations or others who do not report traditional risk factors for infection.[3] In particular, potential clusters involving two or more cases with a common health care procedure during the likely exposure period should immediately be reported to public health authorities. Likewise, a single case of acute hepatitis B or C (or documented seroconversion) occurring in a cancer, hemodialysis, or transplant patient, long-term care resident, or routine blood donor represents a "red flag" for medical transmission that deserves thorough investigation.

PREVENTING HEALTH CARE–ASSOCIATED BLOODBORNE VIRUS INFECTIONS

Outbreaks have occurred in a variety of health care settings and affected differing patient populations. A common thread, however, is that they were all devastating to the patients who were impacted, damaged public trust in health care institutions, and ultimately resulted from the failure of providers to understand and follow the most basic concepts of injection safety and infection control.[66] The CDC and other groups have published best practice guidance to prevent health care–associated infections and to assist facilities in risk assessment and investigation of identified breaches in infection control.[36,60] Awareness, understanding, and implementation of these recommendations all remain suboptimal. These trends and findings point to the need for a multifaceted approach focusing on surveillance, oversight, enforcement, safety engineered technologies, and continued education efforts aimed at ensuring safe injection practices in all health care settings.

Efforts toward enforcement of basic standards of infection control are being pursued at both the state and federal levels, as illustrated by the following examples. New York State has long required all of its licensed health care professionals to undergo training in infection control and barrier precautions at the time their license is obtained and every 4 years thereafter.[67] New Jersey requires that outpatient endoscopy and other surgical centers retain the services of a licensed infection control professional.[68] New York and Nevada have recently increased licensing, accreditation, and inspection requirements for physician offices and clinics that perform procedures that involve certain levels of anesthesia or sedation.[69,70] At the federal level, CMS has recently begun to incorporate expanded infection control requirements into its Conditions for Coverage for outpatient settings including hemodialysis and ambulatory surgical centers.[35,71] With assistance from the CDC, CMS has also provided infection control guidance, including information on injection and medication safety, to surveyors for use during facility inspections.[71]

In addition to enforcement strategies, there are still many opportunities and needs for targeted educational initiatives. The continued occurrence of outbreaks, such as those described in this article, highlight a lack of awareness and understanding by health care providers of issues related to injection safety and infection control and indicate an urgent need for improved education at all levels of health care delivery. This includes attention to professional curricula at nursing and medical schools to ensure appropriate investments in basic knowledge of infection transmission and prevention, and to vocational training for other health professionals who likewise need to have a clear understanding of basic infection prevention requirements. Ongoing reinforcement of training is equally important and could benefit from periodic certification requirements, such as those implemented at many state health departments to ensure that restaurant food-handlers are appropriately trained. Examples of available resources to assist providers are listed in **Box 4**.

The CDC is working with states and other partners to develop sufficient plans to respond to outbreaks of disease caused in part by the reuse of syringes in outpatient settings and to ensure that infection control measures are adhered to broadly, including provider education and patient awareness activities. As part of this effort, the Safe Injection Practices Coalition, a broad-based group of national health care leaders, was established in 2008. This coalition is working to raise awareness and knowledge of safe injection practices among the public and health care providers through its "One and Only" campaign.

Box 4
Injection safety and related infection control resources

The Centers for Disease Control and Prevention

Injection Safety Website: http://www.cdc.gov/ncidod/dhqp/injectionsafety.html

Division of Healthcare Quality Promotion: http://www.cdc.gov/ncidod/dhqp/index.html

Division of Viral Hepatitis: http://www.cdc.gov/ncidod/diseases/hepatitis/

Safe Injection Practices Coalition One and Only Campaign

http://www.oneandonlycampaign.org

The World Health Organization Safe Injection Global Network

http://www.who.int/injection_safety/en/

SUMMARY

Recent increases in the reported number of HBV and HCV outbreaks and related incidents involving breakdowns in basic infection control have exposed tens of thousands of patients to needless risks and undermined trust in the health care system. This trend must be reversed. It is critical that medical professionals and others recognize the responsibility of all health care providers to implement safe care practices, the need for strengthened public health surveillance, and the importance of enhanced infection control education. With the spotlight now being directed at this issue, health care providers everywhere need to pause, with their staff and colleagues, to review injection procedures and other aspects of care to ensure that safe practices are understood and followed by all.

REFERENCES

1. Shepard CW, Simard EP, Finelli L, et al. Hepatitis B virus infection: epidemiology and vaccination. Epidemiol Rev 2006;28:112–25.
2. Shepard CW, Finelli L, Alter MJ. Global epidemiology of hepatitis C virus infection. Lancet Infect Dis 2005;5:558–67.
3. Williams IT, Perz JF, Bell BP. Viral hepatitis transmission in ambulatory health care settings. Clin Infect Dis 2004;38:1592–8.
4. Thompson ND, Perz JF, Moorman AC, et al. Nonhospital health care–associated hepatitis B and C virus transmission: United States, 1998–2008. Ann Intern Med 2009;150:33–9.
5. Prati D. Transmission of hepatitis C virus by blood transfusion and other medical procedures: a global review. J Hepatol 2006;24:607–16.
6. Busch MP, Kleinman SH, Nemo GJ. Current and emerging infectious risks of blood transfusions. JAMA 2003;289:959–62.
7. Centers for Disease Control and Prevention (CDC). Transmission of hepatitis B and C viruses in outpatient settings—New York, Oklahoma, and Nebraska, 2000–2002. MMWR Morbid Mortal Weekly Rep 2003;52:901–6.
8. Allos BM, Schaffner W. Transmission of hepatitis B in the health care setting: the elephant in the room…or the mouse? J Infect Dis 2007;195:1245–7.
9. Centers for Disease Control and Prevention (CDC). Acute hepatitis C virus infections attributed to unsafe injection practices at an endoscopy clinic—Nevada, 2007. MMWR Morbid Mortal Weekly Rep 2008;57:513–7.
10. Moore ZS, Schaefer M, Thompson N, et al. Hepatitis C virus infections associated with myocardial infusion studies, North Carolina, 2008. Presented at Annual Scientific Meeting of the Society for Healthcare Epidemiology, San Diego (CA), March 21, 2009.
11. State of New Jersey Department of Health and Senior Services. Hepatitis B Outbreak Investigation. Available at: http://www.nj.gov/health/hepb_investigation.shtml. Accessed November 13, 2009.
12. Maki DG, Crnich CJ. History forgotten is history relived: nosocomial infection control is also essential in the outpatient setting. Arch Intern Med 2005;165:2565–7.
13. Jarvis WR. Infection control and changing health-care delivery systems. Emerg Infect Dis 2001;7:170–3.
14. Alter M. Healthcare should not be a vehicle for transmission of hepatitis C virus. J Hepatol 2008;48:2–4.
15. Mortimer PP. Away with multi-use vials! AIDS 1999;13(13):1779–81.

16. Hughes RR. Syringe contamination following intramuscular and subcutaneous injections. J R Army Med Corps 1946;87:156–68.
17. Evans RJ, Spooner ETC. A possible mode of transfer of infection by syringes used for mass inoculation. Br Med J 1950;2:185–8.
18. Fleming A, Oglivie AC. Syringe needles and mass inoculation technique. Br Med J 1951;1:543–6.
19. Lutz CT, Bell CE Jr, Wedner HJ, et al. Allergy testing of multiple patients should no longer be performed with a common syringe. N Engl J Med 1984;310:1335–7.
20. Koepke JW, Reller LB, Masters HA, et al. Viral contamination of intradermal skin test syringes. Ann Allergy 1985;55:776–8.
21. Trépanier CA, Lessard MR, Brochu JG, et al. Risk of cross-infection related to the multiple use of disposable syringes. Can J Anaesth 1990;37:156–9.
22. Plott RT, Wagner RF Jr, Tyring SK. Iatrogenic contamination of multidose vials in simulated use: a reassessment of current patient injection technique. Arch Dermatol 1990;126:1441–4.
23. Druce JD, Locarnini SA, Birch CJ. Isolation of HIV-1 from experimentally contaminated multidose local anaesthetic vials. Med J Aust 1995;162(10):513–5.
24. Apetrei C, Becker J, Metzger M, et al. Potential for HIV transmission through unsafe injections. AIDS 2006;20:1074–6.
25. Comstock RD, Mallonee S, Fox JL, et al. A large nosocomial outbreak of hepatitis C and hepatitis B among patients receiving pain remediation treatments. Infect Control Hosp Epidemiol 2004;25(7):576–83.
26. New York State Department of Health. Nassau County and State Health Departments alert 36 patients to infection control error by Long Island doctor. Albany (NY). 2008. Available at: http://www.health.state.ny.us/press/releases/2008/2008-01-15_health_department_alerts_patients_to_infection_control_error.htm. Accessed June 17, 2009.
27. Kent County Health Department. Kent County Health Department to notify additional patients of potential risks. Grand Rapids (MI). 2007. Available at: http://www.accesskent.com/NewsRoom/PressReleases/2007/2007_Stokes.htm. Accessed June 17, 2009.
28. Thompson ND, Perz JF. Eliminating the blood: ongoing outbreaks of hepatitis B virus infection and the need for innovative glucose monitoring technologies. J Diabetes Sci Technol 2009;3:283–8.
29. US Food and Drug Administration (FDA). Risk of transmission of blood-borne pathogens from shared use of insulin pens: information for healthcare professionals. FDA alert. 2009. Available at: http://www.fda.gov/Drugs/DrugSafety/PostmarketDrugSafetyInformationforPatientsandProviders/DrugSafetyInformationforHeathcareProfessionals/ucm133352.htm. Accessed June 17, 2009.
30. Sonoki K, Yoshinari M, Iwase M, et al. Regurgitation of blood into insulin cartridges in the pen-like injectors. Diabetes Care 2001;24:603–4.
31. Macedo de Oliveira A, White KL, Leschinsky DP, et al. An outbreak of hepatitis C virus infections among outpatients at a hematology/oncology clinic. Ann Intern Med 2005;142:898–902.
32. Wenzel RP, Edmond MB. Patient-to-patient transmission of hepatitis C virus. Ann Intern Med 2005;142:940–1.
33. Bennett SN, McNeil MM, Bland LA, et al. Postoperative infections traced to contamination of an intravenous anesthetic, propofol. N Engl J Med 1995;333:147–54.

34. Grohskopf LA, Roth VR, Feikin DR, et al. Serratia liquefaciens bloodstream infections from contamination of epoetin alfa at a hemodialysis center. N Engl J Med 2001;344:1491–7.
35. Centers for Disease Control and Prevention (CDC). Infection control requirements for dialysis facilities and clarification regarding guidance on parenteral medication vials. MMWR Morb Mortal Wkly Rep 2008;57(32):875–6.
36. Centers for Disease Control and Prevention (CDC). Guideline for isolation precautions: preventing transmission of infectious agents in healthcare settings 2007. Atlanta (GA): US Department of Health and Human Services. CDC; 2007. Available at: http://www.cdc.gov/ncidod/dhqp/gl_isolation.html. Accessed November 13, 2009.
37. Samandari T, Malakmadze N, Balter S, et al. A large outbreak of hepatitis B virus infections associated with frequent injections at a physician's office. Infect Control Hosp Epidemiol 2005;26:745–50.
38. Centers for Disease Control and Prevention (CDC). Recommendations for preventing transmission of infections among chronic hemodialysis patients. MMWR Morb Mortal Wkly Rep 2001;50(No. RR-5):1–43.
39. Flaum A, Malmros H, Preston E. Eine nosocomiale ikterus-epedemie. Acta Med Scand 1926;(Suppl 1):544–53.
40. Polish LB, Shapiro CN, Bauer F, et al. Nosocomial transmission of hepatitis B virus associated with a spring-loaded fingerstick device. N Engl J Med 1992;326:721–5.
41. Centers for Disease Control and Prevention (CDC). Nosocomial hepatitis B virus infections associated with reusable fingerstick blood sampling devices—Ohio and New York City, 1996. MMWR Morbid Mortal Weekly Rep 1997;46:217–21.
42. Khan AJ, Cotter SM, Schulz B, et al. Nosocomial transmission of hepatitis B virus infection among residents with diabetes in a skilled nursing facility. Infect Control Hosp Epidemiol 2002;23:313–8.
43. Centers for Disease Control and Prevention (CDC). Transmission of hepatitis B virus among persons undergoing blood glucose monitoring in long-term care facilities—Mississippi, North Carolina and Los Angeles County, California, 2003–2004. MMWR Morbid Mortal Weekly Rep 2005;54:220–3.
44. Patel AS, White-Comstock MB, Woolard CD, et al. Infection control practices in assisted living facilities: a response to hepatitis B outbreaks. Infect Control Hosp Epidemiol 2009;30:209–14.
45. Deline CR. Opening our eyes to healthcare associated hepatitis [electronic letter] 2009. Available at: http://www.annals.org/content/150/1/33.abstract. Accessed November 13, 2009.
46. Louie RF, Lau MJ, Lee JH, et al. Multicenter study of the prevalence of blood contamination on point-of-care glucose meters and recommendations for controlling contamination. Point Care 2005;4:158–63.
47. Bond WW, Favero MS, Petersen NJ, et al. Survival of hepatitis B virus after drying and storage for one week. Lancet 1981;1(8219):550–1.
48. Kamili S, Krawczynski K, McCaustland K, et al. Infectivity of hepatitis C virus in plasma after drying and storing at room temperature. Infect Control Hosp Epidemiol 2007;28:519–24.
49. Froio N, Nicastri E, Comandini UV, et al. Contamination by hepatitis B and C viruses in the dialysis setting. Am J Kidney Dis 2003;42:546–50.
50. Girou E, Chevaliez S, Challine D, et al. Determinant roles of environmental contamination and noncompliance with standard precautions in the risk of hepatitis C virus transmission in a hemodialysis unit. Clin Infect Dis 2008;47:627–33.

51. Centers for Disease Control and Prevention (CDC). Hepatitis C Virus transmission at an outpatient hemodialysis unit—New York, 2001–2008. MMWR Morb Mortal Wkly Rep 2009;58:189–94.

52. Thompson ND, Novak RT, Datta D, et al. Hepatitis C virus (HCV) transmission in the hemodialysis setting: the importance of infection control practices and aseptic technique. Infect Control and Hosp Epidemiol 2009;30:900–3.

53. Fissell RB, Bragg-Gresham JL, Woods JD, et al. Patterns of hepatitis C prevalence and seroconversion in hemodialysis units from three continents: the DOPPS. Kidney Int 2004;65:2335–42.

54. Forns X, Martinez-Bauer E, Feilu A, et al. Nosocomial transmission of HCV in the liver unit of a tertiary care center. Hepatology 2005;41:115–22.

55. Thompson ND, Hellinger WC, Kay RS, et al. Healthcare-associated hepatitis C virus transmission among patients in an abdominal organ transplant center. Transpl Infect Dis 2009;11:324–9.

56. Centers for Disease Control and Prevention (CDC). Guidelines for environmental infection control in health-care facilities. Recommendations of CDC and the Healthcare Infection Control Practices Advisory Committee (HICPAC). MMWR Recomm Rep 2003;52(RR-10):1–42.

57. Rutala WA, Weber DJ. The Healthcare Infection Control Practices Advisory Committee (HICPAC). Guideline for disinfection and sterilization in healthcare facilities, 2008. Available at: http://www.cdc.gov/ncidod/dhqp/pdf/guidelines/Disinfection_Nov_2008.pdf. Accessed June 18, 2009.

58. ASGE Standards of Practice Committee. Banerjee S, Shen B, et al. Infection control during GI endoscopy. Gastrointest Endosc 2008;67:781–90.

59. Seoane-Vazquez E, Rodriguez-Monguio R, Visaria J, et al. Endoscopy-related infections and toxic reactions: an international comparison. Endoscopy 2007; 39:742–78.

60. Patel PR, Srinivasan A, Perz JF. Developing a broader approach to management of infection control breaches in health care settings. Am J Infect Control 2008;36: 685–90.

61. Nelson DB. Hepatitis C virus cross-infection during endoscopy: is it the tip of the iceberg or the absence of ice? Gastrointest Endosc 2007;65:589–91.

62. Muscarella LF. The risk of disease transmission associated with inadequate disinfection of gastrointestinal endoscopes. J Hosp Infect 2006;63:345–7.

63. House Veterans' Affairs Committee. Oversight and investigations subcommittee. Endoscopy procedures at the VA: what happened, what has changed?. Washington, DC. 2009. Available at: http://veterans.house.gov/hearings/hearing.aspx?newsid=417. Accessed November 13, 2009.

64. Nelson DB, Jarvis WR, Rutala WA, et al. Multi-society guidelines for reprocessing flexible gastrointestinal endoscopes. Infect Control Hosp Epidemiol 2003;24(7): 532–7.

65. Centers for Disease Control and Prevention (CDC). Surveillance for acute viral hepatitis—United States, 2007. MMWR Morb Mortal Wkly Rep 2009;58(no. SS-3):1–27.

66. Allen M. Poll finds ill feelings on health care. Las Vegas Sun. 2008. Available at: http://www.lasvegassun.com/news/2008/may/27/poll-finds-ill-feelings-health-care/. Accessed November 13, 2009.

67. New York State Department of Health. Health care provider infection control training. Albany (NY). Available at: http://www.health.state.ny.us/professionals/diseases/reporting/communicable/infection/hcp_training.htm. Accessed June 17, 2009.

68. Maher AC, Hohf BA, Kassai MA, et al. Affiliation of infection prevention professionals: a model for improving infection control in ambulatory care settings. Am J Infect Control 2006;34:E144–5.

69. New York State Department of Health. Health care professionals & patient safety: office-based surgery. Available at: http://www.health.state.ny.us/professionals/office-based_surgery/. Accessed June 17, 2009.

70. State of Nevada. Assembly bill no. 123–committee on health and human services. Available at: http://www.leg.state.nv.us/75th2009/Bills/AB/AB123_EN.pdf. Accessed June 19, 2009.

71. Center for Medicaid and State Operations/Survey and Certification Group. State Operations Manual (SOM) Appendix L, Ambulatory Surgical Centers (ASC) Comprehensive. Revision Baltimore (MD). 2009. Available at: http://www.cms.hhs.gov/SurveyCertificationGenInfo/downloads/SCLetter09_37.pdf. Accessed June 19, 2009.

Health Care Workers as Source of Hepatitis B and C Virus Transmission

Abigail L. Carlson, BA[a], Trish M. Perl, MD, MSc[a,b,c,*]

KEYWORDS

- Hepatitis B • Hepatitis C • Nosocomial transmission
- Health care worker

Hepatitis B virus (HBV) and hepatitis C virus (HCV) are endemic worldwide, with prevalence varying geographically. This group of infections remains a major global cause of morbidity and mortality. More than 2 billion people have been infected with HBV alone,[1] whereas HCV has infected an estimated 170 million people worldwide.[2]

The prevalence of HBV varies enormously, from 0.1% to more than 20%,[1] depending on the vaccination strategies of the country or region in question. In North America, the prevalence varies from less than 2% to 15%.[3] Similarly, the prevalence of HCV infection in North America ranges between 0.2% and 18% of the general population.[4]

Health care–associated transmission of viral hepatitis has been well documented in the literature.[5–9] Among these, HBV and HCV are of greatest importance, not only due to the morbidity and mortality associated with these infections but also because, in their chronic phase, infected persons can transmit to others via blood and other infected secretions, with implications for the patients and for the management of infected providers. In 2000, the World Health Organization estimated that 60,000 occupationally acquired HBV and 16,000 occupationally acquired HCV infections occurred among health care workers (HCWs).[10] Although patient-to-provider and patient-to-patient transmission are most often described, an important subset of cases involves the transmission of infection from ill providers to their patients. This article reviews known cases of HCW-to-patient transmission of HBV and HCV, appropriate infection

[a] Department of Hospital Epidemiology and Infection Control, The Johns Hopkins Hospital, 425 Osler, 600 North Wolfe Street, Baltimore, MD 21287, USA
[b] Division of Infectious Diseases, Department of Medicine, Johns Hopkins University School of Medicine, 425 Osler, 600 North Wolfe Street, Baltimore, MD 21287, USA
[c] Department of Epidemiology, Johns Hopkins University Bloomberg School of Public Health, 425 Osler, 600 North Wolfe Street, Baltimore, MD 21287, USA
* Corresponding author. Department of Hospital Epidemiology and Infection Control, Johns Hopkins Hospital, 425 Osler, 600 North Wolfe Street, Baltimore, MD 21287.
E-mail address: tperl@jhmi.edu (T.M. Perl).

Clin Liver Dis 14 (2010) 153–168
doi:10.1016/j.cld.2009.11.003
1089-3261/10/$ – see front matter © 2010 Elsevier Inc. All rights reserved.
liver.theclinics.com

prevention and control measures to limit nosocomial spread, and issues surrounding management of the infected provider.

HEALTH CARE WORKER–TO–PATIENT TRANSMISSION OF HEPATITIS B

Subsequent to hepatitis B testing becoming available in the early 1970s, at least 52 reported HBV-infected HCWs have been implicated in transmission of their infection to more than 500 patients (**Table 1**).[11–20] The last reported case of provider-to-patient transmission of HBV occurred in the United Kingdom in 2001, which, it is important to note, was after implementation of universal vaccination of HCWs.[17]

Published transmission rates for HCW-to-patient transmission range from 0.2% to 13%, with even higher transmission rates associated with certain categories of invasive procedures involving increased risk of blood and body fluid exposure.[11,12,20,21] HCWs performing these types of procedures, such as dentists and surgeons, account for the majority of transmissions to patients. The largest group of HCWs associated with provider-to-patient HBV transmission is surgeons, with 38 surgeons documented as a source of infection in patients. These include obstetricians, gynecologists, general surgeons, cardiothoracic surgeons, and orthopedists. Transmission has been demonstrated from HCWs in a variety of occupations, however, including a respiratory therapist,[22] two cardiac pump technicians,[23,24] an electroencephalography technician,[19] and a general practitioner.[25] Additionally, procedures, such as coronary artery bypass, valve replacement, hysterectomy, and cesarean section, which require blind or digital suturing, involve restricted anatomic spaces, or entail poor visualization of a site where sharp instruments are used, are more likely to be associated with transmission of hepatitis viruses because of increased risk of percutaneous injury to a HCW.[11,12,26]

One other group of HCWs, HBV-infected dentists and oral surgeons, accounted for the majority of provider-to-patient transmissions in the 1970s and early 1980s, although no recent transmissions from dentists or oral surgeons have been reported.[12] Among the possible explanations for the lack of transmission from this group in recent years are the more widespread espousal of standard (formerly universal) precautions, including routine glove use, in dental and oral surgery practices and the increased immunity in dental HCWs themselves resulting from HBV vaccination.[12,27]

In settings where hepatitis B vaccination has been widely implemented, reported rates of transmission have decreased. Still, inadequate infection control practices— including the failure to use gloves where there is a possibility of exposure to blood— have been identified as a risk factor for transmission in many cases.[16,23,28–33] This includes the failure to use gloves when there is contact with blood or body fluids or during procedures with a risk of blood and body fluid exposure and failure to double glove during surgical procedures. In one example, an electroencephalography technician implicated in HBV transmission did not use gloves while providing patient care despite frequent use of reusable subdermal electrodes.[19] In other cases, compromised skin integrity of providers' hands has likely contributed to transmission. Some infected surgeons have described the routine observance of blood on their hands when removing gloves after an operation without visible tears in the gloves.[28,32] Surgeons have reported lesions on the tips of their index fingers after prolonged suturing or can recreate bleeding by simulating suture tying, showing paper cut–like injuries after 1 hour.[13,32] As part of one simulation with an HBV-infected provider, investigators used molecular typing to document the feasibility of transmission by showing that hepatitis B surface antigen (HbsAg) was found on the exterior surface of a surgeon's

Table 1
Health care worker-to-patient HBV transmission, 1996 to present

Country	Publication	Year of Index Case	Health Care Worker Occupation	Hepatitis Be Antigen Status	Hepatitis Be Antigen-Negative Precore Mutant	Provider Hepatitis B Virus DNA Level (Copies/mL)
United Kingdom	The Incident Control Teams, 1996	1992	Cardiothoracic surgeon	+	NA	NA
	The Incident Investigation Teams, 1997[a]	1988	General surgeon	−	Yes	1×10^7 copies/mL
	The Incident Investigation Teams, 1997	1993	Obstetrician/gynecologist	−	Yes	4.4×10^6 copies/mL
	The Incident Investigation Teams, 1997	1994	Obstetrician/gynecologist	−	Yes	5.5×10^6 copies/mL
	The Incident Investigation Teams, 1997	1995	General Surgeon/urologist	−	Yes	2.5×10^5 copies/mL
	Sundkvist et al, 1998	1996	Orthopedic surgeon	−	Yes	NA
	Oliver et al, 1999	1993–1994	General surgeon	+	NA	NA
	Molyneaux et al, 2000	1999	Cardiothoracic surgeon	−	Yes	1×10^6 copies/mL
	Laurenson et al, 2007	2001	Surgeon	−	No	$>1 \times 10^6$ copies/mL
United States	Harpaz et al, 1996[a]	1992	Cardiothoracic surgeon	+	NA	1×10^9 copies/mL
Canada	Hepatitis B outbreak investigation team, 2000	Unspecified	Electroencephalogram technician	+	NA	NA
Netherlands	Spijkerman et al, 2002	1998	General surgeon	+	NA	5×10^9 g Eq/mL

Abbreviations: NA, data not available; +, antigen positive; −, antigen negative.
[a] Included in data from Bell DM, Shapiro CN, Ciesielski CA, et al. Preventing bloodborne pathogen transmission from health-care workers to patients. The CDC perspective. Surg Clin North Am 1995;75(6):1189–203.

gloves.[26,32,34] Other compromises to skin integrity reported in the literature include bleeding warts, exudative and eczematous dermatitis, and frequent, vigorous scrubbing of the hands.[22,23,29,31] Such lessons are important considerations in countries with developing and developed health care systems, as focus on low-cost infection prevention measures in low and high endemic settings can lead to significant patient protection.

The stage and infectivity of the provider's HBV infection also seem to play a significant role in HCW-to-patient transmission. In particular, the presence of hepatitis B e antigen (HBeAg) in a provider's serum has been strongly correlated with risk of transmission. Until 1988, for all cases where HBeAg status of the HCW was known, only HBeAg-positive providers had been implicated in transmission of infection to their patients. Starting that year, however, public health officials in the United Kingdom began to report cases of HCW-to-patient transmission involving HBeAg-negative providers.[16] Since then, seven HBeAg-negative HCWs have been documented as transmitting their infection to patients.[15–18] Six of those seven HCWs were infected with a "precore" variant strain of HBV that prevented production of the e antigen.[35] This particular infection is commonly reported in Asia and its role in nosocomial HBV transmission needs to be carefully monitored. Furthermore, it has implications for guidelines and policies regarding management of HBV-infected HCWs (discussed later).

HEALTH CARE WORKER–TO–PATIENT TRANSMISSION OF HEPATITIS C

Transmission of HCV has been reported from 17 HCWs to more than 300 patients (**Table 2**).[2,11,36–50] In addition, investigations into potential provider-to-patient HCV transmission in the United States are ongoing. Published rates of transmission from infected HCWs to patients range from 0.04% to 0.48%[47,49] but may be higher among HCWs associated with intravenous drug use. Many of the factors associated with increased HCW-to-patient transmission that have been characterized in the literature on HBV also apply HCV transmission. Several patients infected by HCV-positive HCWs underwent an exposure-prone procedure (EPP) or a high-risk procedure performed by the implicated HCW, including cesarean section,[49] hysterectomy,[38] coronary artery replacement,[41] valve replacement,[43] and hip arthroplasty.[47] Infection control violations included the failure of the HCW to routinely use gloves in all contacts with risk of exposure to blood or body fluid of the patient[37,45–47] and surgeons not routinely double gloving during procedures.[49] Compromised skin integrity of providers' hands has again also been associated with transmission. An open and weeping wound on an anesthesiology assistant's hand was thought to be the route of acquisition and transmission in one case from Germany,[48] whereas in the case from France, the HCW had a history of atopic dermatitis.[45] In two of the reported cases, analyses of genetic relatedness between HCV strains in HCWs and patients indicated that the HCW in question became infected from occupational exposures involving an HCV-positive patient, then subsequently infected other susceptible patients, forming a chain of patient-to-provider-to-patient transmission.[37,48] Similar series of transmissions have also been reported in the literature on hepatitis B.[22,52]

One relationship that has emerged in HCV transmission from HCWs to patients that has not been seen in reports on HBV is the link to intravenous drug use by an infected HCW.[36,44,50,53] This includes HCWs self-administering patient narcotics and analgesics before injecting patients with the same needle.[50,53] The occupations of the involved HCWs reflect access to narcotics and include anesthesiologists,[44,50] nurse anesthetists,[36] and surgical technicians.[53]

Table 2
Provider-to-patient hepatitis C virus transmission, 1992 to present

Country	Year Index Case Identified	Health Care Worker Occupation	Number of Infected Patients (Published Transmission Rate)	Provider Hepatitis C Virus RNA Level	Risk Factors Identified
United States	1991	Outpatient surgical technician	Approximately 40	NA	IVDU
	1996	Anesthesiologist	1	3.79×10^7 g Eq/mL	NA
	2001	Cardiothoracic surgeon	3	NA	EPPs
	2004	Nurse anesthetist	15	NA	Possible IVDU
United Kingdom	1994	Cardiothoracic surgeon	1 (0.36%)	NA	EPPs
	1999	Obstetrician/gynecologist	8	NA	EPPs
	1999	Unspecified (surgical team member)	2	NA	EPPs
	1999	Cardiac surgeon	1	NA	NA
	Unspecified	Anesthesiologist	1	1.1×10^7 copies/mL	NA
Germany	1998	Anesthesiology assistant	5	1×10^6 copies/mL	Weeping wound on hand, irregular glove use
	1999	Orthopedic surgeon	1 (0.48%)	1.3×10^6 IU/mL	EPPs
	2000	Obstetrician/gynecologist	1 (0.04%)	2.66×10^5 IU/mL	EPPs, irregular double gloving for procedures
	2001	Anesthesiologist	3	7.34×10^6 IU/mL	Irregular glove use, inadequate disinfectants
Spain	1992–1994	Cardiothoracic surgeon	5	2.2×10^7 g Eq/mL	EPPs
	1998	Anesthesiologist	Approximately 275	NA	IVDU
France	1996	Unspecified	1	NA	EPPs, atopic eczema
Israel	2003	Anesthesiologist	33	10^5 copies/mL	IVDU

Abbreviations: IVDU, intravenous drug use; NA, data not available.
Data compiled from Refs. [2,11,36-51]

PRACTICES TO PREVENT TRANSMISSION OF BLOOD-BORNE PATHOGENS FROM INFECTED HEALTH CARE WORKERS

Although all HCWs are expected to observe standard precautions (previously called universal precautions) during patient care, failures are commonly reported (discussed previously). These precautions advocate frequent hand hygiene and the appropriate use of protective barriers, such as gloves, masks, eye protection and faces shields, and gowns when there is a possibility of exposure to blood, blood-containing fluids, or other infectious body fluids (eg, cerebrospinal fluid, semen, vaginal secretions, and peritoneal fluid).[54] A recent literature review of health care–associated HBV and HCV transmission outside of acute care hospitals in the United States described 33 outbreaks in the past decade: 12 in outpatient settings, 6 in hemodialysis centers, and 15 in long-term care facilities.[55] Although this reflects patient-to-patient transmission in most cases, the putative mechanism of transmission in all cases was a failure of personnel to follow standard and other fundamental infection control precautions. Similarly, the number of HBV and HCV HCW-to-patient transmissions where these precautions were not observed and the decline in dentist-to-patient HBV transmissions after their widespread adoption in dental practice highlight the importance of these straightforward measures in preventing transmission of these blood-borne pathogens. Finally, given the number of incidents related to HCWs with weeping or exudative dermatitis, recommendations to have HCWs with such conditions limit or cease all direct patient care activities and refrain from contact with any equipment that may be used in patient care until such time as their dermatitis has resolved should be entertained.[33]

Several professional societies and governmental bodies have developed supplemental guidelines for HBV- and HCV-infected HCWs (**Table 3**). In addition to the importance of standard precautions, these guidelines recommend the use of double gloves during all procedures for providers who are HBV or HCV infected.[26] A Cochrane review from 2006 examining 31 randomized controlled trials highlights why this latter recommendation is important. Fourteen studies compared the number of perforations in single gloves versus innermost double gloves during operations with techniques that, in theory, pose a low risk for HCW injury.[62] Even in these low-risk situations, pooled analyses of these studies results revealed that perforations of the single glove were fourfold (odds ratio 4.10; 95% CI, 3.30–5.09) more likely than perforations to the innermost double glove. Five studies evaluated the proportion of perforations detected intraoperatively by the wearer. Surgical staff wearing single gloves identified 21% (71 of the 192) of perforations, whereas staff wearing two sets of gloves (double gloving) identified 77% (193 of 225) of perforations intraoperatively (odds ratio 0.08; 95% CI, 0.04–0.17). As the investigators acknowledge, the quality of the primary studies examining these questions remains poor, and additional studies directly examining the infection prevention and control value of various gloving systems are needed. Nonetheless, the cumulative evidence continues to suggest that double gloving should be a routine practice in all surgical procedures and that the use of a double glove system may aide in recognition of perforation events, thus avoiding potential exposures in HCWs and patients.

MANAGEMENT OF INFECTED HEALTH CARE WORKERS
Screening for Hepatitis B and C Infection in Health Care Workers

Screening HCWs for hepatitis B and C remains a complex and controversial issue, and significant variation exists between the North American, British, and European approaches. In the United States, the Centers for Disease Control and Prevention (CDC) and the Society for Healthcare Epidemiology of America (SHEA) provide the

Table 3
Guidelines for management of hepatitis B virus– and hepatitis C virus–infected health care workers

	United States	Canada	United Kingdom	Europe
Screening and vaccination				
No mandatory screening for HBV or HCV	X	X		
Mandatory screening for HBV and HCV in HCWs performing EPPs			X	
HBV vaccination of HCWs	X	X	X	X
Additional HBV vaccine dose for anti-HBs levels of 10–100 mIU/mL after three-dose series			X	X
Universal vaccination program in place	X	X		N/A
Management of infected health care workers				
Restrictions based on HBeAg status			X	X
Referral to expert committee based on HBeAg status	X	X		
Restrictions based on HBV DNA levels			X	X
Restrictions based on HCV RNA			X	
Patient notification				
Patient notification of provider seropositivity in absence of known transmission	X			

Abbreviation: N/A, not applicable.
Data compiled from Refs.[51,56–61]

most comprehensive guidance. SHEA is currently in the process of updating its recommendations for management of the infected HCW. In some cases, CDC and SHEA recommendations overlap, although they differ on certain key issues. Neither recommends mandatory testing of HCWs for HBsAg or anti-HCV antibody.[26,33] Voluntary testing for hepatitis B for those HCWs engaged in exposure-prone procedures (EPPs) is, however, suggested, and these HCWs are generally considered ethically obligated to know their HBsAg antibody status and their HBeAg status if they are HBsAg positive.[33,63] Testing for these serologic markers is also recommended in instances of HCW exposure to blood, blood-containing fluid, or other infectious body fluids. At this time, neither SHEA nor the CDC has endorsed HCV screening for HCWs performing EPPs.

Canadian guidelines do not mandate screening of HCWs for HBV or HCV but emphasize the ethical responsibility of those HCWs performing EPPs to know their HBsAg and anti-HCV antibody status.[56] Additionally, routine screening for serologic markers of infection in HBV vaccine nonresponders is advocated.

European countries, in contrast, have more aggressively screened HCWs. In the United Kingdom, HCWs who perform EPPs must be screened for HBsAg and anti-HCV.[57,58] Italian guidelines for HCV are similar to those of the United Kingdom in requiring testing for providers performing invasive procedures, whereas German HCV guidelines require HCV testing for all HCWs on employment with repeat testing at regular intervals.[2]

In addition, all HCWs whose work may expose them to blood or infectious body fluids and who also have a previous history of hepatitis B vaccination should be tested for anti–hepatitis B surface antibody (anti-HBs). Documentation of anti-HBs status identifies those providers who have not mounted an immune response to vaccination and require a second vaccination series or further screening for HBsAg, and it facilitates the proper management of these HCWs.

Hepatitis B Virus Vaccination

Hepatitis B vaccine became available in the United States in 1982, at which time the CDC's Advisory Committee on Immunization Practices recommended routine HBV vaccination for HCWs. This US immunization strategy contributed to the large declines in the rate of HBV infection among HCWs during the 1980s and 1990s.[59] Currently, the CDC recommends that all HCWs who are negative for anti-HBs and are at risk for contact with blood or body fluid be vaccinated against hepatitis B with the standard three-dose vaccination series.[64] Serum anti-HBs titers should be obtained a minimum of 1 to 2 months after vaccination to demonstrate antibody response. Those HCWs who fail to develop titers greater than 10 mIU/mL after one series are given a second series of vaccine; the chance of an immunologic response after the second series is 30% to 50%.[64,65] All HCWs who have been vaccinated for hepatitis B and have no measurable immunologic response should be tested for HBsAg, as chronic infection is a known cause of vaccination failure. At least five cases of HBV transmission from provider to patient have involved previously vaccinated HCWs who failed to demonstrate appropriate responses to partial or complete courses of vaccine.[12,17] Whether or not these HCWs acquired their HBV infection before or after vaccination remains unclear.

Hepatitis B vaccination is also required of HCWs in the United Kingdom and Canada and is recommended by the European Consensus Group on HBV and HCV infections in health care workers.[51,60,61] The guidelines of the Canadian Consensus Conference on Infected Health Care Workers are similar to those of the CDC and recommend vaccination of all HCWs without evidence of anti-HBs who are at risk for contact with blood and body fluids and postvaccination screening for those HCWs not responding to vaccine.[56] Canadian guidelines also propose that vaccination be mandatory for all HCWs who perform EPPs and that all vaccine nonresponders and HCWs with contraindications to vaccination undergo screening for infection with HBV on a routine basis.

UK and European Consensus Group guidelines contain a more detailed algorithm for management of HBV vaccine nonresponders. UK guidelines recommend that individuals who have completed the HBV vaccination series and have anti-HBs titers between 10 mIU/mL and 100 mIU/mL receive an immediate, additional one-time dose of vaccine.[60] Anti-HBs titers do not need to be rechecked to demonstrate further response. European guidelines vary based on whether or not a HCW performs EPPs.[51] In both groups, HCWs with anti-HBs levels of 10 to 100 mIU/mL receive a supplementary dose of vaccine. In contrast to UK guidelines, they recommend that antibody response be confirmed using an alternative assay. Testing for HBsAg is not recommended, however, for HCWs who do not perform EPPs. For those HCWs who do perform EPPs, HBsAg testing is recommended for all providers who fail to demonstrate anti-HBs levels above 100 mIU/mL.

The United States and Canada have instituted universal, population-based vaccination programs for hepatitis B.[59,61] In each of these countries, the rates of hepatitis B infection have declined among those age groups affected by the universal vaccination programs. During the 1990s, the Advisory Committee on Immunization Practices additionally recommended that children and adolescents (ages 0–18) who were not vaccinated as infants receive hepatitis B vaccination. It is as yet unclear whether or not these trends will lead to decreasing numbers of HBV-infected HCWs and patients.

Hepatitis B e Antigen and Serum Hepatitis B Virus DNA

HBeAg is associated with increased infectivity and elevated serum levels of viral DNA in chronic HBV infection. The presence of antibody to hepatitis e antigen (anti-HBe) correlates with lower levels of HBV DNA and a corresponding decline in infectivity. In the cases of provider-to-patient HBV transmission for which provider HBeAg status is known, the vast majority involves HBeAg-positive HCWs. Until recently, HBeAg was used as the sole serologic marker of transmission risk in infected HCWs. Since the 1990s, however, reports of HBV transmission from seven HBeAg-negative HCWs to patients have altered the approach[15–18] and led to an increased focus on the use of viral load as a more appropriate indicator of risk. Despite general agreement that viral load should be incorporated into the national and even international approach to such patients, debate continues on the appropriate threshold for placing restrictions on HBV-infected providers. In a study of the sera from six of the seven HBeAg-negative HCWs, measurements of HBV DNA levels varied between 4.0×10^4 g Eq/mL and 1.5×10^9 g Eq/mL, although all serum samples were drawn at least 3 months after the documented transmissions.[35] All six HCWs were also found to be infected with the precore variant of hepatitis B that results from a mutation in codon 28 of the precore/core gene that prevents production of HBeAg. No correlation was demonstrated between infection with precore variants and HBV DNA levels in the control group of the study, although in certain HCWs infected with a precore variant, viral loads were of levels typically observed in HBeAg-positive individuals. The seventh transmitting HBeAg-negative HCW, who was not included in this study, had a documented HBV DNA level of greater than 10^6 g Eq/mL but was not infected with a precore variant.[17] HBV DNA levels for an HBeAg-positive general surgeon and an HBeAg-positive cardiothoracic surgeon implicated in provider-to-patient transmission are also reported in the literature, showing elevated viral loads of 5.0×10^9 g Eq/mL and 1.0×10^9 g Eq/mL, respectively.[13,32]

Current CDC and Canadian guidelines recommend that a panel of experts advise HBeAg-positive providers who perform EPPs on whether or not and under what circumstances they may continue to practice (discussed later).[33,56] SHEA recommends that HBeAg-positive HCWs refrain from performing "activities that have been identified epidemiologically as associated with a risk for provider-to-patient HBV transmission despite the use of appropriate infection control procedures."[26] As yet, none of these groups has restricted the activities of HCWs based on serum HBV DNA levels. UK guidelines are more conservative and require that a HBV-infected HCW who performs EPPs be HBeAg-negative and have HBV DNA levels less than 10^3 g Eq/mL.[57] The Netherlands has established a cutoff of 10^5 g Eq/mL for determining whether or not an infected HCW may perform EPPs, regardless of HBeAg status.[21,51] The European Consensus Group guidelines leave the determination of a threshold value to individual nations but recommend using 10^4 g Eq/mL as an appropriate compromise between risk of transmission and the loss of highly-trained providers.[51]

Exposure-prone Procedures

Although many of the international guidelines share features and themes, defining operations that are associated with transmission has been challenging. As discussed previously, certain gynecologic, cardiothoracic, and orthopedic procedures have been frequently linked to provider-to-patient transmission with HBV and HCV. In addition to these and other epidemiologically associated procedures, many guidelines currently in place use the category of EPPs to help delineate the restrictions placed on HBV- and HCV-positive providers. The definition of EPPs, however, is often vague, and consensus regarding the most appropriate definitions has not been achieved. In its 1991 recommendations on preventing HIV and HBV transmission to patients during EPPs, the CDC described EPPs as those involving "digital palpation of a needle tip in a body cavity or the simultaneous presence of the HCW's fingers and a needle or other sharp instrument or object in a poorly visualized or highly confined anatomic site" where "performance of [these] procedures presents a recognized risk of percutaneous injury to the HCW, and—if such injury occurs—the HCW's blood is likely to contact the patient's body cavity, subcutaneous tissues, and/or mucous membranes."[33] Beyond listing those procedures already linked to blood-borne pathogen transmission, however, regulatory agencies have refrained from labeling specific procedures as exposure prone. This has allowed local public health authorities, professional organizations, and institutions to develop their own classifications. In 1992, Dr William Roper, then director of the CDC, informed state and territorial health departments that the categorization of EPPs should be determined "on a case-by-case basis, taking into consideration the specific procedure as well as the skill, technique and possible impairment of the infected health care worker."[12]

The Canadian guidelines define EPPs as "procedures during which transmission of HBV, HCV or HIV from a HCW to patients is most likely to occur," including repair of major traumatic injuries and major cutting of oral or perioral tissue in addition to operations identified by the CDC.[56] The guidelines also acknowledge that classification of EPPs is challenging and state that the definition of EPPs provided is intended to guide practitioners and expert panels as they consider they details of an individual case.

Guidelines issued by the United Kingdom define EPPs as "those invasive procedures where there is a risk that injury to the worker may result in exposure of the patient's open tissues to the blood of the worker."[57] These guidelines define EPPs as do the CDC and Canadian guidelines but also include prehospital trauma care and care of patients where the HCW is exposed to a regular risk of biting. Furthermore, they expand their definition to better characterize low-risk procedures, stating that "[p]rocedures where the hands and fingertips of the worker are visible and outside the patient's body at all times, and internal examinations or procedures that do not involve possible injury to the worker's gloved hands from sharp instruments and/or tissues, are considered not to be exposure prone."

Like the definitions themselves, the restrictions placed on HBV- and HCV-infected HCWs who wish to perform EPPs vary between countries. Guidelines for HBV-infected HCWs are generally more complete than those for HCV-infected providers, and many nations do not have explicit policies addressing HCWs known to be infected with hepatitis C.[2] Those guidelines that do exist for HCV-infected HCWs tend to be less restrictive. In the United States, there are no absolute prohibitions for providers known to be infected with HBV or HCV.[26,33,66] HBV-infected HCWs who are also HBeAg positive and wish to perform EPPs must be advised individually by an expert review panel (discussed previously) and may have their practice restricted based on the recommendations of the panel. Guidelines developed by the American College of Surgeons follow the CDC in allowing HVB- and HCV-infected HCWs to perform EPPs.[63] SHEA guidelines, however, recommend that HCWs with HBeAg be restricted from those procedures that have been linked to previous HCW-to-patient HBV transmission.[26] They additionally advise that those HCWs who are epidemiologically implicated in provider-to-patient transmission cease the practice of EPPs. Because most cases of HCV transmission from infected providers were reported after the SHEA guidelines were published, the guidelines do not currently place any restrictions on health care providers infected with hepatitis C unless implicated in HCW-to-patient transmission. SHEA guidelines, however, are currently being updated and may change to reflect the understanding of provider-to-patient HCV transmission that has developed over the past decade.

Canadian guidelines, like those of the CDC, do not forbid HBV- and HCV-infected providers outright from performing EPPs, but they require that, on learning of any positive test for a blood-borne pathogen, those HCWs do not practice such procedures until reviewed by an expert panel.[56] This recommendation applies to HCWs who are HBsAg positive and HBeAg positive and those who are HCV infected. HCWs who perform or will perform EPPs but decline screening are assumed to be HBeAg positive and should be managed according to the guidelines for HBeAg-positive providers.

As discussed previously, all HCWs in the United Kingdom who are HBsAg and HBeAg positive are forbidden from performing EPPs, regardless of HBV DNA levels.[58] Providers who are HBsAg positive but do not produce HBeAg must be tested for viral load. Those providers with viral loads of greater than 10^3 g Eq/mL are restricted in the same manner as HBeAg-positive HCWs. HCWs with viral loads of 10^3 g Eq/mL or less are permitted to perform EPPs but must be retested every 12 months and are subject to restrictions once their HBV DNA level surpasses 10^3 g Eq/mL. In contrast to US and Canadian guidelines, any HCW in the United Kingdom actively infected with hepatitis C with detectable HCV RNA levels is barred from performance of EPPs.[57] All individuals training for careers in which EPPs form a significant portion of the work must be tested for hepatitis C antibodies and, if positive, HCV RNA. Any individual found to have detectable HCV RNA levels is restricted from undertaking training for such professions. Those individuals who receive antiviral therapy and maintain a response to treatment for 6 months after cessation of therapy (ie, undetectable serum HCV RNA), may resume their practice of EPPs or training for such procedures, although they must also be retested after a second 6-month interval to prove a sustained response.

Germany is one of the few countries that incorporate variations in HCV RNA concentrations into their guidelines for HCV-positive HCWs. German guidelines state that HCWs who are infected with hepatitis C but have a serum HCV RNA less than 1×10^3 IU/mL may practice without restrictions.[2] Those providers with serum concentrations of HCV RNA between 1×10^3 IU/mL and 1×10^5 IU/mL are referred to an expert panel, who determine what constraints, if any, are placed on an infected provider's practice. Any provider with HCV RNA concentrations above 1×10^5 IU/mL is prohibited from the performance of any EPP.

Patient Notification of Provider Hepatitis B Virus and Hepatitis C Virus Status

One of the most controversial aspects of the 1991 CDC guidelines for HBV-positive providers who perform EPPs was the requirement that HBsAg- and HBeAg-positive HCWs disclose their serologic status to any patient undergoing such procedures.[33] Although the response of professional organizations to this position has been varied, most organizations agree that such disclosure produces more harm than benefit. The SHEA position paper on management of HCWs infected with blood-borne pathogens states, "such a disclosure very likely would require an HCW to abandon healthcare work," and that given what was known of the transmission risks from infected providers, such measures were unjustified.[26] The one exception given is when the patient has been exposed to the HCWs blood or blood-containing fluids; thus, the benefit to the patient of disclosure clearly outweighs harm to the provider. Even in these cases, this guideline emphasizes the need for protecting the confidentiality of the HCW to the extent that is feasible. A revision of these guidelines is under way, however, that will likely reflect the new technology and data that have emerged in the last 10 years. The American Medical Association (AMA) does not have a specific position regarding disclosure to patients of seropositivity in HBV- or HCV-infected HCWs, although AMA policy for HIV-positive physicians specifies that "the confidentiality of the HIV-infected physician should be protected as with any HIV patient; and [k]nowledge of the health care worker's HIV serostatus should be restricted to those few professionals who have a medical need to know."[67] As the 1991 CDC guidelines were written to apply to HIV- and HBV-infected workers, the AMA's stance on the issue is in direct contradiction to aforementioned CDC requirement. State health departments seem to have taken a similar position to professional societies and, since 1992, when states were charged with adopting the CDC guidelines or developing their own "equivalent" policies, most states have opted to refrain from requiring disclosure of seropositivity in an infected HCW to patients undergoing EPPs.[12,26,56]

The Canadian Consensus Conference on Infected Health Care Workers holds a position similar to that of US organizations.[56] Their guidelines do not recommend the disclosure of a HCW's positive serostatus to patients undergoing EPPs given the known risks of transmission from infected providers. However, they except those situations in which patients have been exposed to the blood of an infected HCW, although, as with US guidelines, they stress that the HCW implicated in those situations does not need to be identified to the patient by name. The European Consensus Group does not address the issue of whether or not disclosure should be made to patients but does propose that, as far as HBV is concerned, if such a disclosure is made voluntarily by a provider, the provider ought to be permitted to continue the performance of EPPs regardless of HBeAg positivity or HBV viral load.[51]

SUMMARY

HBV and HCV are rarely reported in the literature, although many transmissions remain unreported. Although HCW vaccination has led to significant decreases in transmissions in North America and Europe, HCWs in other parts of the world remain at risk for acquisition and transmission of hepatitis B and C. The management of HBV- and HCV-infected health care providers will continue to pose a complex challenge as we enter the next decade. As options for treatment develop further and the epidemiology of these diseases changes over time, practices must respond accordingly. Moreover, the movement of patients and providers across borders has added new dimensions to understanding and management of viral hepatitis transmission in the health care setting[68] and has emphasized the international importance of national universal vaccination programs. With increased vaccination, due vigilance in observation of infection control measures, proper guidance for those HCWs infected with HBV and HCV, and further understanding of the spread of hepatitis B and C in the health care setting, the transmission of these viruses from providers to those under their care will hopefully remain a rarity.

REFERENCES

1. World Health Organization. Hepatitis B. Geneva: Department of Communicable Diseases Surveillance and Response, World Health Organization; 2002. Available at: http://www.who.int/csr/disease/hepatitis/HepatitisB_whocdscsrlyo2002_2.pdf. Accessed August 6, 2009.
2. Raggam RB, Rossmann AM, Salzer HJ, et al. Health care worker-to-patient transmission of hepatitis C virus in the health care setting: many questions and few answers. J Clin Virol 2009. DOI:10.1016/j.jcv.2009.04.015.

3. Carey WD. The prevalence and natural history of hepatitis B in the 21st century. Cleve Clin J Med 2009;76(Suppl 3):S2–5.
4. World Health Organization. Hepatitis C. Geneva: Department of Communicable Diseases Surveillance and Response, World Health Organization; 2002. Available at: http://www.who.int/csr/disease/hepatitis/Hepc.pdf. Accessed August 6, 2009.
5. Jensenius M, Ringertz SH, Berild D, et al. Prolonged nosocomial outbreak of hepatitis A arising from an alcoholic with pneumonia. Scand J Infect Dis 1998; 30(2):119–23.
6. Lettau LA, Alfred HJ, Glew RH, et al. Nosocomial transmission of delta hepatitis. Ann Intern Med 1986;104(5):631–5.
7. Siddiqui A, Jooma R, Smego J, et al. Nosocomial outbreak of hepatitis E infection in Pakistan with possible parenteral transmission. Clin Infect Dis 2005;40(6): 908–9.
8. Lanini S, Puro V, Lauria F, et al. Patient to patient transmission of hepatitis B virus: a systematic review of reports on outbreaks between 1992 and 2007. BMC Med 2009;7(1):15.
9. Sánchez-Tapias J. Nosocomial transmission of hepatitis C virus. J Hepatol 1999; 31(Suppl 1):107–12.
10. Prüss-Ustün A, Rapiti E, Hutin Y. Estimation of the global burden of disease attributable to contaminated sharps injuries among health-care workers. Am J Ind Med 2005;48(6):482–90.
11. Puro V, Scognamiglio P, Ippolito G. [Trasmissione di HIV, HBV o HCV da operatore sanitario infetto a paziente]. Med Lav 2003;94(6):556–68 [in Italian].
12. Bell DM, Shapiro CN, Ciesielski CA, et al. Preventing bloodborne pathogen transmission from health-care workers to patients. The CDC perspective. Surg Clin North Am 1995;75(6):1189–203.
13. Spijkerman IJ, van Doorn LJ, Janssen MH, et al. Transmission of hepatitis B virus from a surgeon to his patients during high-risk and low-risk surgical procedures during 4 years. Infect Control Hosp Epidemiol 2002;23(6):306–12.
14. Heptonstall J. Lessons from two linked clusters of acute hepatitis B in cardiothoracic surgery patients. Commun Dis Rep CDR Rev 1996;6(9):R119–25.
15. Sundkvist T, Hamilton GR, Rimmer D, et al. Fatal outcome of transmission of hepatitis B from an e antigen negative surgeon. Commun Dis Public Health 1998;1(1):48–50.
16. Transmission of hepatitis B to patients from four infected surgeons without hepatitis B e antigen. Incident Investigation Teams and Others. N Engl J Med 1997; 336(3):178–84.
17. Laurenson IF, Jones DG, Hallam NF, et al. Transmission of hepatitis B virus from a vaccinated healthcare worker. J Hosp Infect 2007;66(4):393–4.
18. Molyneaux P, Reid TM, Collacott I, et al. Acute hepatitis B in two patients transmitted from an e antigen negative cardiothoracic surgeon. Commun Dis Public Health 2000;3(4):250–2.
19. An outbreak of hepatitis B associated with reusable subdermal electroencephalogram electrodes. Hepatitis B outbreak investigation team. CMAJ 2000;162(8): 1127–31.
20. Oliver SE, Woodhouse J, Hollyoak V. Lessons from patient notification exercises following the identification of hepatitis B e antigen positive surgeons in an English health region. Commun Dis Public Health 1999;2(2):130–6.
21. Buster EH, van der Eijk AA, Schalm SW. Doctor to patient transmission of hepatitis B virus: implications of HBV DNA levels and potential new solutions. Antiviral Res 2003;60(2):79–85.

22. Snydman DR, Hindman SH, Wineland MD, et al. Nosocomial viral hepatitis B: a cluster among staff with subsequent transmission to patients. Ann Intern Med 1976;85(5):573–7.
23. Coutinho RA, Albrecht-van Lent P, Stoutjesdijk L, et al. Hepatitis B from doctors. Lancet 1982;319(8267):345–6.
24. Heptonstall J. Outbreaks of hepatitis B virus infection associated with infected surgical staff. Commun Dis Rep CDR Rev 1991;1(8):R81–5.
25. Grob PJ, Bischof B, Naeff F. Cluster of hepatitis B transmitted by a physician. Lancet 1981;318(8257):1218–20.
26. Management of healthcare workers infected with hepatitis B virus, hepatitis C virus, human immunodeficiency virus, or other bloodborne pathogens. AIDS/TB Committee of the Society for Healthcare Epidemiology of America. Infect Control Hosp Epidemiol 1997;18(5):349–63.
27. Kohn WG, Collins AS, Cleveland JL, et al. Guidelines for infection control in dental health-care settings–2003. MMWR Recomm Rep 2003;52(RR-17):1–61.
28. Carl M, Blakey DL, Francis DP, et al. Interruption of hepatitis B transmission by modification of a gynaecologist's surgical technique. Lancet 1982;1(8274):731–3.
29. Reingold AL, Kane MA, Murphy BL, et al. Transmission of hepatitis B by an oral surgeon. J Infect Dis 1982;145(2):262–8.
30. Hadler SC, Sorley DL, Acree KH, et al. An outbreak of hepatitis B in a dental practice. Ann Intern Med 1981;95(2):133–8.
31. Shaw FE Jr, Barrett CL, Hamm R, et al. Lethal outbreak of hepatitis B in a dental practice. JAMA 1986;255(23):3260–4.
32. Harpaz R, Von Seidlein L, Averhoff FM, et al. Transmission of hepatitis B virus to multiple patients from a surgeon without evidence of inadequate infection control. N Engl J Med 1996;334(9):549–54.
33. Centers for Disease Control and Prevention. Recommendations for preventing transmission of human immunodeficiency virus and hepatitis B virus to patients during exposure-prone invasive procedures. MMWR Recomm Rep 1991; 40(RR-8):1–9.
34. Harpaz R, Von Seidlein L, Averhoff F, et al. Hepatitis B virus transmission associated with cardiothoracic surgery. Infect Control Hosp Epidemiol 1994;15(5):352.
35. Corden S, Ballard AL, Ijaz S, et al. HBV DNA levels and transmission of hepatitis B by health care workers. J Clin Virol 2003;27(1):52–8.
36. Roche WF. Nurse accused of spreading hepatitis C at military hospital. Los Angeles Times 2008. Available at: http://articles.latimes.com/2008/mar/12/nation/na-nurse12. Accessed July 15, 2009.
37. Cody SH, Nainan OV, Garfein RS, et al. Hepatitis C virus transmission from an anesthesiologist to a patient. Arch Intern Med 2002;162(3):345–50.
38. Public Health Laboratory Service. Two hepatitis C lookback exercises—national and in London. Commun Dis Rep CDR Wkly 2000;10(14):125–8.
39. Brown P. Surgeon infects patient with hepatitis C. BMJ 1999;319(7219):1219.
40. Public Health Laboratory Service. Hepatitis C lookback exercise. Commun Dis Rep CDR Wkly 2000;10(23):203–6.
41. Duckworth GJ, Heptonstall J, Aitken C. Transmission of hepatitis C virus from a surgeon to a patient. Commun Dis Public Health 1999;2(3):188–92.
42. Mawdsley J, Teo CG, Kyi M, et al. Anesthetist to patient transmission of hepatitis C virus associated with non exposure-prone procedures. J Med Virol 2005;75(3):399–401.
43. Esteban JI, Gomez J, Martell M, et al. Transmission of hepatitis C virus by a cardiac surgeon. N Engl J Med 1996;334(9):555–61.

44. Shemer-Avni Y, Cohen M, Keren-Naus A, et al. Iatrogenic transmission of hepatitis C virus (HCV) by an anesthesiologist: comparative molecular analysis of the HCV-E1 and HCV-E2 hypervariable regions. Clin Infect Dis 2007;45(4):e32–8.

45. Lot F, Delarocque-Astagneau E, Thiers V, et al. Hepatitis C virus transmission from a healthcare worker to a patient. Infect Control Hosp Epidemiol 2007; 28(2):227–9.

46. Stark K, Hanel M, Berg T, et al. Nosocomial transmission of hepatitis C virus from an anesthesiologist to three patients—epidemiologic and molecular evidence. Arch Virol 2006;151(5):1025–30.

47. Ross RS, Viazov S, Roggendorf M. Phylogenetic analysis indicates transmission of hepatitis C virus from an infected orthopedic surgeon to a patient. J Med Virol 2002;66(4):461–7.

48. Ross RS, Viazov S, Gross T, et al. Transmission of hepatitis C virus from a patient to an anesthesiology assistant to five patients. N Engl J Med 2000;343(25):1851–4.

49. Ross RS, Viazov S, Thormahlen M, et al. Risk of hepatitis C virus transmission from an infected gynecologist to patients: results of a 7-Year retrospective investigation. Arch Intern Med 2002;162(7):805–10.

50. Bosch X. Hepatitis C outbreak astounds Spain. Lancet 1998;351(9113):1415.

51. Gunson RN, Shouval D, Roggendorf M, et al. Hepatitis B virus (HBV) and hepatitis C virus (HCV) infections in health care workers (HCWs): guidelines for prevention of transmission of HBV and HCV from HCW to patients. J Clin Virol 2003;27(3):213–30.

52. Garibaldi RA, Rasmussen CM, Holmes AW, et al. Hospital-acquired serum hepatitis: report of an outbreak. JAMA 1972;219(12):1577–80.

53. Sehulster L, Taylor J, Hendricks K, et al. Hepatitis C outbreak linked to narcotic tampering in an ambulatory surgical center. In: Abstracts of the 1997 Interscience Conference on Antimicrobial Agents and Chemotherapy. Washington, DC: American Society for Microbiology Press; 1997. p. 293.

54. Centers for Disease Control and Prevention. Update: universal precautions for prevention of transmission of human immunodeficiency virus, hepatitis B virus, and other bloodborne pathogens in health-care settings. MMWR Morb Mortal Wkly Rep 1988;37(24):377–82, 387–8.

55. Thompson ND, Perz JF, Moorman AC, et al. Nonhospital health care-associated hepatitis B and C virus transmission: United States, 1998–2008. Ann Intern Med 2009;150(1):33–9.

56. Health Canada. Proceedings of the consensus conference on infected health care worker risk for transmission of bloodborne pathogens. Can Commun Dis Rep 1998;24(Suppl 4): i, iii, 1–25; i–iii, 1–28.

57. UK Department of Health. Hepatitis C infected health care workers. Health Services Circular 2002/010. UK Department of Health; 14 August 2002. Available at: http://www.dh.gov.uk/en/Publicationsandstatistics/Lettersandcirculars/Healthservicecirculars/index.htm. Accessed July 26, 2009.

58. UK Department of Health. Hepatitis B infected health care workers. Health Services Circular 2000/020. UK Department of Health; 23 June 2000. Available at: http://www.dh.gov.uk/en/Publicationsandstatistics/Lettersandcirculars/Healthservicecirculars/index.htm. Accessed July 26, 2009.

59. Centers for Disease Control and Prevention. Hepatitis B vaccination—United States, 1982–2002. MMWR Morb Mortal Wkly Rep 2002;51(25):549–63.

60. U.K. Department of Health. Hepatitis B. In: Salisbury D, Ramsay M, Noakes K, editors. Immunisation against infectious disease. London: Stationary Office; 2006. p. 161–84.

61. National Advisory Committee on Immunization. Hepatitis B Vaccine. In: Canadian immunization guide. Ottowa (Canada): Public Health Agency of Canada; 2006. p. 189–204.
62. Tanner J, Parkinson H. Double gloving to reduce surgical cross-infection. Cochrane Database Syst Rev 2006;(3):CD003087.
63. American College of Surgeons. Statement on the surgeon and hepatitis. Bull Am Coll Surg 1999;84(4):2–24.
64. U.S. Public Health Service. Updated U.S. Public Health Service Guidelines for the Management of Occupational Exposures to HBV, HCV, and HIV and Recommendations for Postexposure Prophylaxis. MMWR Recomm Rep 2001;50(RR-11): 1–52.
65. Hadler S, Francis D, Maynard J, et al. Long-term immunogenicity and efficacy of hepatitis B vaccine in homosexual men. N Engl J Med 1986;315(4):209–14.
66. Recommendations for prevention and control of hepatitis C virus (HCV) infection and HCV-related chronic disease. Centers for Disease Control and Prevention. MMWR Recomm Rep 1998;47(RR-19):1–39.
67. American Medical Association. Guidance for HIV-Infected Physicians and other Health Care Workers. AMA PolicyFinder 2008(I-08):H-20.912. Available at: http://www.ama-assn.org/ama/no-index/advocacy/11760.shtml. Accessed July 20, 2009.
68. Harling R, Turbitt D, Millar M, et al. Passage from India: an outbreak of hepatitis B linked to a patient who acquired infection from health care overseas. Public Health 2007;121(10):734–41.

Management of Acute Hepatitis C

Anurag Maheshwari, MD[a], Paul J. Thuluvath, MD, FRCP[a,b],*

KEYWORDS

- Hepatitis C • Interferon • Intravenous drug use
- Sustained virological response

The World Health Organization[1] estimates that about 170 million people (3% of the world's population) are infected with hepatitis C virus (HCV), with the highest prevalence in Egypt and the lowest in Sweden. Blood transfusions from unscreened donors and unsafe therapeutic procedures are the major modes of HCV transmission in the developing world. Although injection drug use accounts for the vast majority of newly diagnosed HCV infections in the developed countries, its impact in the developing countries is unclear because of a paucity of data. Acute infection with HCV leads to symptomatic hepatitis in only a minority of patients, and recent studies suggest that spontaneous clearance of virus is higher in symptomatic acute hepatitis C infection. Pooled data from various studies suggest that higher sustained viral clearance rates could be achieved with a shorter course of antiviral treatment in the early stages of chronic HCV infection. This article examines the diagnosis of acute infection and critically appraises the various treatment regimens.

DIAGNOSIS OF ACUTE HCV INFECTION

An accurate diagnosis of acute HCV infection can often be elusive. The most accepted method of diagnosis is the documentation of recent (ie, in the previous 6 months) seroconversion of HCV antibody associated with detectable HCV RNA and elevated liver enzymes. These stringent diagnostic criteria can only be fulfilled during the follow-up of a documented needle-stick exposure or by prospective surveillance of high-risk groups, such as injection drug users. When these criteria are not met, additional circumstantial evidence to support the diagnosis may be considered. This evidence includes documented exposure to HCV, high levels of alanine aminotransferase (ALT; >10–20 times the upper limit of normal), exclusion of other causes of acute liver

[a] Institute for Digestive and Liver Diseases, Mercy Medical Center, 301 St Paul's Place, POB suite 718, Baltimore, MD 21202, USA

[b] Department of Surgery & Medicine, Georgetown University School of Medicine, Washington, DC, USA

* Corresponding author. Department of Surgery & Medicine, Georgetown University School of Medicine, Washington DC.

E-mail address: thuluvath@gmail.com (P.J. Thuluvath).

Clin Liver Dis 14 (2010) 169–176
doi:10.1016/j.cld.2009.11.007
1089-3261/10/$ – see front matter © 2010 Published by Elsevier Inc.

liver.theclinics.com

disease and autoimmune hepatitis, and increasing numbers of reactive proteins on the recombinant immunoblot assay (RIBA) on follow-up testing.[2] However, acute exacerbation of chronic HCV infection or other conditions, such as alcoholic hepatitis and drug-induced liver dysfunction, are confounding factors that could sometimes make a diagnosis of acute HCV hepatitis difficult.

HCV RNA detection by polymerase chain reaction (PCR) in a previously HCV-RNA–negative patient remains the most sensitive and specific method of diagnosing an acute HCV infection. Detectable viremia usually occurs within 2 weeks after HCV exposure, but viral titers may fluctuate during an acute infection. Therefore, testing is recommended using the newer PCR methodologies that have extremely low limits of detection at 5 to 15 IU/mL. Detection of viremia followed by the development of HCV antibody is highly suggestive of an acute HCV infection. HCV antibody detection by conventional enzyme-linked immunosorbent assay (ELISA) testing is not always reliable. The development of anti-HCV antibodies usually occurs between 2 to 6 months after acute exposure and may be delayed further in the immunosuppressed populations. Some studies have suggested that HCV antibody response may lag behind the onset of symptoms in 30% of patients,[3] making the test unreliable for the diagnosis of acute HCV infection in a patient with symptomatic hepatitis. Similarly, the RIBA test is also not sensitive for the diagnosis of acute HCV infection, although some authors have suggested that an increase in the number of reactive bands on follow-up testing may be used as corroborative evidence of acute HCV seroconversion.[2] Testing for anti-HCV IgM levels is no longer performed, because it is not indicative of acute infection and its titers remain fairly constant after seroconversion.[4]

There are no specific guidelines for postexposure surveillance of HCV infection. The Centers for Disease Control and Prevention recommendations include measurement of HCV antibodies (Ab) and ALT at baseline, HCV RNA by PCR at 4 to 6 weeks after exposure, and HCV Ab and ALT activity at 4 to 6 months.[5] There are no accepted guidelines, however, for monitoring patients with detectable viremia after an acute infection. It has been suggested that HCV RNA is measured every 4 weeks after an acute infection, because viral titers may fluctuate or even become undetectable during the first year of infection. Continued serial HCV-RNA monitoring is also recommended for those patients who are believed to have had spontaneous viral clearance, because late relapses may occur and could be missed if testing is discontinued prematurely.

TREATMENT OF ACUTE HCV INFECTION

Unlike the treatment of chronic HCV infection, the published studies show considerable heterogeneity with regard to trial design (randomized vs nonrandomized), inclusion criteria (type of exposure and methods of diagnosis), patient characteristics, treatment introduction relative to exposure date or onset of symptoms, and treatment modality (varying schedules of interferon [IFN] and ribavirin doses and durations). This makes it harder to make firm recommendations or provide a specific algorithm for the care of patients with acute HCV infection.

Although there were no large, multicenter, controlled trials, 2 meta-analyses have demonstrated that the treatment of patients with acute HCV infection is beneficial and cost-effective.[6,7] These pooled data suggested that higher rates of sustained virological response (SVR) could be achieved with a shorter duration of therapy, and moreover, patients with acute HCV hepatitis tolerated IFN treatment very well with low rates of dropout. Despite the increasing evidence of efficacy, however, there is no consensus on the optimal timing of treatment, the treatment duration and regimen, and the role of therapy for patients with coexistent HIV infection or end-stage renal disease.

OPTIMAL TIMING OF TREATMENT

Although treatment of acute HCV infection is highly effective, the immediate introduction of treatment is not recommended for all patients, especially those with symptomatic infection, because many of them may undergo spontaneous viral clearance. The goal of therapy is to avoid treatment in those patients who are more likely to undergo spontaneous viral clearance and treat others when treatment is likely to be most effective.

The incidence of spontaneous clearance of HCV infection is highest among patients with symptomatic HCV hepatitis. Two recent German studies of patients with acute HCV infection found higher rates of spontaneous viral clearance among those with symptomatic hepatitis (67% and 52%), and in one of these studies, spontaneous viral clearance was not observed among asymptomatic patients.[8,9] The time to viral clearance was 34.7 ± 22.1 days from the onset of symptoms in one of the studies,[8] and in the other study, all patients demonstrating spontaneous clearance had undetectable HCV-RNA levels at 4 months from the onset of symptoms.[9] The presence of symptoms, such as jaundice, in these patients may suggest a robust antiviral cellular immunity that leads to higher rates of spontaneous viral clearance. Other recent studies have suggested that spontaneous clearance occurred in up to 23% of asymptomatic patients, and usually this occurred within 14 weeks of seroconversion.[10] In these studies, spontaneous clearance was seen more often among young patients and women and those with jaundice, symptomatic hepatitis, or non-genotype 1 HCV infection.

Early studies with standard IFN therapy recommended immediate establishment of therapy for acute hepatitis C infection because of the excellent treatment responses.[11] However, later observations from the German studies suggested that treatment could be avoided in a significant minority of patients by waiting for 12 to 16 weeks from the onset of symptoms. Waiting for 12 weeks did not reduce the SVR rates as shown by one study[12] where 15 of 16 patients who failed to spontaneously clear HCV RNA for 12 weeks responded to antiviral treatment; this suggests that it is prudent to wait for 12 weeks before initiating antiviral treatment, especially when patients present with symptomatic hepatitis C. This strategy may avoid unnecessary treatment of those who are likely to have spontaneous viral clearance. This strategy was examined using 12 weeks of pegylated (PEG)-IFN α-2b (1.5 μg/kg) monotherapy[10] in 129 patients with acute HCV infection who failed to clear the virus spontaneously by week 8, by randomizing them to begin treatment at week 8, 12, or 20. Of the 43 patients in each group, 41 (95%), 40 (93%) and 33 (77%) had SVR when treatment was initiated at week 8, 12, and 20, respectively. This study suggested that the optimal time to initiate therapy might be week 12, because the response rate dropped off sharply in the group that initiated treatment at week 20 compared with the other 2 groups. Serious concerns were raised regarding the validity of this study, but this is the only published data to date regarding the optimal timing.

The German network for viral hepatitis (HEP-NET) recently presented their preliminary data (published as an abstract)[13] from a randomized trial that evaluated immediate therapy for asymptomatic patients and immediate versus delayed (12 weeks from onset of symptoms) therapy for those with symptomatic hepatitis. The intent-to-treat analysis suggested lower SVR rates for those undergoing delayed treatment (78% vs 54%), but dropout during the observation phase of the delayed treatment group seemed to be responsible for the difference. The SVR rates remained excellent for those who adhered to therapy in all arms; SVR rates were similar after immediate treatment for symptomatic hepatitis (arm A, n = 36; SVR 87%), delayed treatment for symptomatic hepatitis (arm B, n = 37; SVR 100%), and immediate treatment for asymptomatic hepatitis (arm C, n = 16; SVR 100%).[13] Although this trial confirmed the efficacy of delayed therapy, the investigators suggested that this strategy should only be applied if adherence can be ensured.

These 2 studies showed that delaying treatment for 3 months from the time of diagnosis does not have a negative effect on SVR rates and avoids unnecessary treatment for those patients who may undergo spontaneous viral clearance. There are only limited data on the optimal timing for treatment in asymptomatic patients, and it may not be unreasonable to offer immediate treatment to them, because they are less likely to clear the virus spontaneously.

DURATION OF TREATMENT

The benchmark study using conventional IFN therapy demonstrated an SVR rate of 98% with 24 weeks of therapy.[11] Japanese investigators suggested that a shorter course of daily IFN for 4 weeks was also highly efficacious. They demonstrated viral clearance in 87% with 4 weeks of daily IFN therapy, and reserved 24-week treatment only for the relapsing group, achieving SVR rates of 100%.[14] However, the treatment regimens used in these studies have not been duplicated and with the advent of PEG-IFN, clinicians are more likely to use it than conventional IFN therapy. The earlier studies with PEG-IFN also used 24 weeks of treatment with similar response rates, but a large multicenter German study using PEG-IFN α-2b for 24 weeks demonstrated a significant number of psychiatric side effects resulting in termination of therapy in 7% (6 of 89) and the death of one subject from suicide.[15] A smaller Swiss study also demonstrated poor adherence with high rates of dropout among intravenous drug users.[16]

Several Italian studies have evaluated the efficacy of PEG-IFN α-2b therapy for 12 weeks. They have demonstrated comparable results in 3 published trials showing viral clearance rates of 72% to 74%.[17–19] These studies have demonstrated a dose-response relationship for PEG-IFN α-2b therapy with higher rates of viral clearance by using dosages higher than 1.2 μg/kg/wk. They also suggest that rapid virological response (RVR: negative HCV-RNA by sensitive PCR assays at 4 weeks) could be used as a predictor of viral clearance with 12 weeks of therapy. An ongoing multicenter study in Italy evaluating the efficacy of 12 versus 24 weeks of PEG-IFN α-2b at 1.5μg/kg may provide additional data on the optimal duration of therapy.

There has been only one study[20] that compared different durations of therapy with 131 patients being randomized to receive 8, 12, or 24 weeks of PEG-IFN α-2b monotherapy. This study reported considerably lower rates of viral clearance in the cohort treated for 8 weeks (68%), when compared with the groups treated for 12 weeks (82%), or 24 weeks (91%). Although the difference between the 12- and 24-week treatment groups was not significant, the latter had higher rates of adverse events and treatment discontinuations. Multivariate analysis showed that the presence of symptoms, non-genotype 1, and RVR at week 4 were associated with improved viral clearance.

The studies discussed in this section showed that there are increased rates of adverse events and poor tolerability when treatment is prolonged beyond 12 weeks. Therefore, it could be proposed that patients with genotype 1 who exhibit RVR at week 4 and those with genotypes 2 or 3 could be treated for 12 weeks, whereas all the others should be treated for 24 weeks or longer.

OPTIMAL TREATMENT REGIMEN

There is no consensus on a standardized treatment regimen, mainly because the studies published to date have included heterogeneous patient populations without any direct comparisons between various treatment modalities. Early Japanese studies used IFN-β, whereas the European and American studies have used IFN-α. The dose of conventional IFN used in various studies has also been variable. With the approval of the PEG-IFNs and evidence of improved efficacy in patients with chronic hepatitis C, more recent studies have used PEG-IFN. Although daily induction therapy has been tried,[11] the benefits of such therapy are unproven, and trials comparing daily IFN therapy to weekly PEG-IFN therapy are lacking. There are also no trials comparing the efficacy of PEG-IFN α-2b with PEG-IFN α-2a. The European studies have used PEG-IFN α-2b therapy, whereas there has been just one US study using PEG-IFN α-2a.[21] These studies demonstrated similar efficacy (SVR rate 94%), but direct comparisons cannot be made because of the small numbers of patients and absence of comparative trials. The Italian studies of PEG-IFN α-2b therapy have demonstrated a clear dose-response relationship and showed significantly higher rates of viral clearance with doses higher than 1.33 μg/kg.[17] The more recent German and Egyptian studies have used PEG-IFN α-2b at 1.5 μg/kg without variable dosing. Unlike the treatment of chronic hepatitis C, there seems to be no advantage in a weight-based dose regimen of PEG-IFN α-2b.

There are only limited data on the additional benefit provided by combining ribavirin with PEG-IFN in patients with acute HCV infection. The few studies that used ribavirin found it to be well tolerated, but response rates were not significantly higher than with PEG-IFN monotherapy. An ongoing multicenter study in Italy has randomized patients to either PEG-IFN α-2b monotherapy or combination therapy of PEG-IFN α-2b and ribavirin. This is the first study to assess the potential benefit of combination therapy for the treatment of acute HCV infection, and until the results of this study are known, it is difficult to define the role of combination therapy. Although unproven, intuitively, one could still consider combination therapy for those that are co-infected with HIV or those without RVR in whom a longer duration of therapy may be necessary.

TREATMENT OF HIV–CO-INFECTED OR HEMODIALYSIS PATIENTS

Recent outbreaks of acute HCV infections related to sexual exposure among the MSM (men who have sex with men) populations have been reported from HIV treatment centers in London and Paris. This has prompted a few small single-center trials for the treatment of acute HCV infection among patients with prior HIV infection. Data from these trials suggest that the rate of viral clearance among the HIV co-infected population is lower than that seen in the HCV mono-infected patients. Gilleece and colleagues[22] reported an SVR rate of 59% in a cohort of 27 patients using a strategy of delayed treatment (after an observation period of 12 weeks) and using PEG-IFN with weight-based ribavirin for 24 weeks. Dominguez and colleagues[23] reported an SVR rate of 71% with delayed treatment using PEG-IFN and fixed-dose ribavirin in a cohort of 14 patients that included a higher proportion of non-genotype 1 patients. Vogel and colleagues[24] reported an SVR rate of 61% in a cohort of 36 patients treated immediately after diagnosis, using a variable regimen of PEG-IFN monotherapy or a combination therapy for 24 or 48 weeks. This study did not demonstrate any added benefit of ribavirin to SVR rates, and patients on combination therapy experienced higher rates of anemia. This study suggested that 48 weeks of therapy was better than 24 weeks, with higher rates of viral clearance. The current guidelines, unsubstantiated by objective data from the HCV-HIV international panel,[25] recommend initiation of combination treatment (regimen of PEG-IFN with weight-based ribavirin for 24 weeks) after 12 weeks of diagnosis to allow for spontaneous clearance.

Hemodialysis is another important risk factor for the acquisition of acute HCV infection among patients with end-stage renal disease. Periodic surveillance for HCV infection in the dialysis population may help identify patients with acute seroconversion. There are only limited data on the optimal therapy for acute HCV infection in this population. Ribavirin is relatively contraindicated in end-stage renal disease because of its renal clearance and the consequent risk of severe hemolytic anemia. Small single-center studies have used varying regimes of conventional IFN and PEG-IFN for 12 to 48 weeks with reported rates of SVR that range from 26% to 66%.[26–29] The variability of treatment regimens and durations makes it difficult to draw any firm

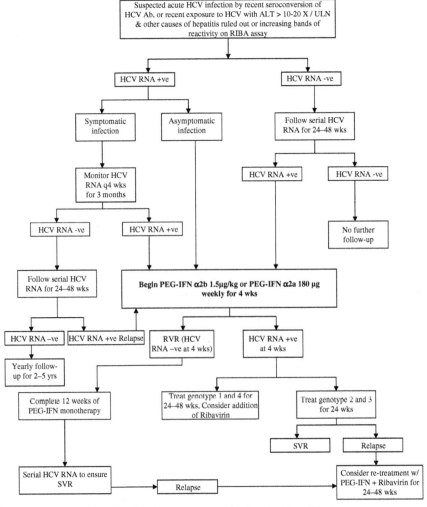

Fig. 1. Treatment algorithm for the management of acute Hepatitis C.

conclusions, and recommendations about treatment of acute HCV infection in the dialysis population remain undefined.

SUMMARY

The identification of acute HCV infection represents a unique window of opportunity for achieving high rates of viral clearance. A waiting period for observation of 12 weeks is recommended for patients with symptomatic hepatitis to allow for spontaneous viral clearance that can occur at high rates in this subgroup. Asymptomatic patients may be treated immediately as they are less likely to undergo spontaneous clearance. Treatment durations could vary from 24 to 48 weeks, but recent data on 12 weeks of treatment are encouraging, especially in those who achieve RVR. Variables that are associated with improved response rates include female gender, presence of symptomatic hepatitis, younger age, non-genotype 1 infection, and RVR. Based on the current data, a management algorithm is proposed (**Fig. 1**) to guide the clinician in making treatment decisions. Certainly, adherence to therapy is extremely important to ensure successful outcomes. The implementation of surveillance programs in high-risk populations, such as injection drug users, patients on hemodialysis, and those with HIV infection, may provide increased opportunities to study the natural history of acute HCV infection and its response to therapy, while reducing the burden of chronic HCV infection.

REFERENCES

1. WHO. Hepatitis C – Global prevalence (update). Wkly Epidemiol Rec 1999;49: 421–8.
2. Wiegand J, Deterding K, Cornberg M, et al. Treatment of acute hepatitis C: the success of monotherapy with (pegylated) interferon alpha. J Antimicrob Chemother 2008;62:860–5.
3. Farci P, Alter HJ, Wong D, et al. A long-term study of hepatitis C virus replication in non-A, non-B hepatitis. N Engl J Med 1991;325:98–104.
4. Quiroga JA, Campillo ML, Catillo I, et al. IgM antibody to hepatitis C virus in acute and chronic hepatitis C. Hepatology 1991;14:38–43.
5. Centers for Disease Control and Prevention. Updated US Public Health Service guidelines for the management of occupational exposures to HBV, HCV, and HIV and recommendations for postexposure prophylaxis. MMWR Morb Mortal Wkly Rep 2001;50(RR-11):1–42.
6. Alberti A, Boccato S, Vario A, et al. Therapy of acute hepatitis C. Hepatology 2002;36:S195–200.
7. Licata A, Di Bona D, Schepis F, et al. When and how to treat acute hepatitis C? J Hepatol 2003;39:1056–62.
8. Hofer H, Watkins-Riedel T, Janata O, et al. Spontaneous viral clearance in patients with acute hepatitis C can be predicted by repeated measurements of serum viral load. Hepatology 2003;37:60–4.
9. Gerlach JT, Diepolder HM, Zachoval R, et al. Acute hepatitis C: high rate of both spontaneous and treatment-induced viral clearance. Gastroenterology 2003;125: 80–8.
10. Kamal SM, Fouly AE, Kamel RR, et al. Peginterferon alfa-2b therapy in acute hepatitis C: impact of onset of therapy on sustained virologic response. Gastroenterology 2006;130:632–8.
11. Jaeckel E, Cornberg M, Wedemeyer H, et al. Treatment of acute hepatitis C with interferon alfa-2b. N Engl J Med 2001;345:1452–7.

12. Santantonio T, Fasano M, Sinisi E, et al. Efficacy of a 24-week course of PEG-interferon alpha-2b monotherapy in patients with acute hepatitis C after failure of spontaneous clearance. J Hepatol 2005;42:329–33.
13. Deterding K, Grüner N, Wiegand J, et al. Early versus delayed treatment of acute Hepatitis C: the German HEP-NET acute HCV-III study – A randomized controlled trial. J Hepatol 2009;50:S380.
14. Nomura H, Sou S, Tanimoto H, et al. Short-term interferon-alfa therapy for acute hepatitis C: a randomized controlled trial. Hepatology 2004;39:1213–9.
15. Wiegand J, Buggisch P, Boecher W, et al. Early monotherapy with pegylated interferon alpha-2b for acute hepatitis C infection: the HEP-NET acute-HCV-II study. Hepatology 2006;43:250–6.
16. Broers B, Helbling B, Francois A, et al. Swiss Association for the Study of the Liver (SASL 18). Barriers to interferon-alpha therapy are higher in intravenous drug users than in other patients with acute hepatitis C. J Hepatol 2005;42:323–8.
17. De Rosa FG, Bargiacchi O, Audagnotto S, et al. Twelve-week treatment of acute hepatitis C virus with pegylated interferon- alpha -2b in injection drug users. Clin Infect Dis 2007;45:583–8.
18. Calleri G, Cariti G, Gaiottino F, et al. A short course of pegylated interferon-alpha in acute HCV hepatitis. J Viral Hepat 2007;14:116–21.
19. De Rosa FG, Bargiacchi O, Audagnotto S, et al. Dose-dependent and genotype-independent sustained virological response of a 12 week pegylated interferon alpha-2b treatment for acute hepatitis C. J Antimicrob Chemother 2006;57:360–3.
20. Kamal SM, Moustafa KN, Chen J, et al. Duration of peginterferon therapy in acute hepatitis C: a randomized trial. Hepatology 2006;43:923–31.
21. Corey KE, Ross AS, Wurcel A, et al. Outcomes and treatment of acute hepatitis C virus infection in a United States population. Clin Gastroenterol Hepatol 2006;4:1278–82.
22. Gilleece YC, Browne RE, Asboe D, et al. Transmission of hepatitis C virus among HIV-positive homosexual men and response to a 24-week course of pegylated interferon and ribavirin. J Acquir Immune Defic Syndr. 2005;40:41–6.
23. Dominguez S, Ghosn J, Valantin MA, et al. Efficacy of early treatment of acute hepatitis C infection with pegylated interferon and ribavirin in HIV-infected patients. AIDS 2006;20:1157–61.
24. Vogel M, Nattermann J, Baumgarten A, et al. Pegylated interferon-alpha for the treatment of sexually transmitted acute hepatitis C in HIV-infected individuals. Antivir Ther 2006;11:1097–101.
25. Soriano V, Puoti M, Sulkowski M, et al. Care of patients coinfected with HIV and hepatitis C virus: 2007 updated recommendations from the HCV-HIV International Panel. AIDS 2007;21:1073–89.
26. Rocha CM, Perez RM, Narciso JL, et al. Interferon-alpha therapy within the first year after acute hepatitis C infection in hemodialysis patients: efficacy and tolerance. Eur J Gastroenterol Hepatol 2007;19:119–23.
27. Al-Harbi AS, Malik GH, Subaity Y, et al. Treatment of acute hepatitis C virus infection with alpha interferon in patients on hemodialysis. Saudi J Kidney Dis Transpl 2005;16:293–7.
28. Griveas I, Germanidis G, Visvardis G, et al. Acute hepatitis C in patients receiving hemodialysis. Ren Fail 2007;29(6):731–6.
29. Gürsoy M, Gür G, Arslan H, et al. Interferon therapy in haemodialysis patients with acute hepatitis C virus infection and factors that predict response to treatment. J Viral Hepat 2001;8:70–7.

Index

Note: Page numbers of article titles are in **boldface** type.

A

Acute liver failure (ALF), 81–82
    oral anti-HBV agents for, 86
Africa
    HBV in, epidemiology of, 6–7
    HCV in, epidemiology of, 12
ALF. See *Acute liver failure (ALF).*
America(s)
    HBV in, epidemiology of, 5–6
    HCV in, epidemiology of, 10–12

B

Blood products, administration of
    HBV transmission related to, 69–70
    HCV transmission related to, 70–71

C

Cancer chemotherapy, chronic HBV due to, 83
Central America, HBV in, epidemiology of, 5–6
Chemotherapy, cancer, chronic HBV due to, 83

D

Dental care, HBV and HCV in, health care–associated transmission of, **93–104**
    described, 95–96
    postexposure prevention, 98–99
Dialysis patients
    HBV in
        management of, 52, 173–175
        natural history of, 50–51
    HBV-related liver disease in, biochemical evidence of, 51–52
    HCV in
        nosocomial transmission of, 53
            modes of, 53–54
        treatment of, 54–56, 173–175

E

Eastern Mediterranean
    HBV in, epidemiology of, 7
    HCV in, epidemiology of, 13
Endoscopy, gastrointestinal, HBV and HCV transmission during, 62–65
    prevention of, 65–66

Clin Liver Dis 14 (2010) 177–183
doi:10.1016/S1089-3261(09)00103-2
1089-3261/10/$ – see front matter © 2010 Elsevier Inc. All rights reserved.

Moving?

Make sure your subscription moves with you!

To notify us of your new address, find your **Clinics Account Number** (located on your mailing label above your name), and contact customer service at:

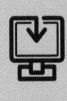

Email: journalscustomerservice-usa@elsevier.com

800-654-2452 (subscribers in the U.S. & Canada)
314-447-8871 (subscribers outside of the U.S. & Canada)

Fax number: 314-447-8029

Elsevier Health Sciences Division
Subscription Customer Service
3251 Riverport Lane
Maryland Heights, MO 63043

*To ensure uninterrupted delivery of your subscription, please notify us at least 4 weeks in advance of move.